MAX YOUR MEMORY
the complete **visual** program

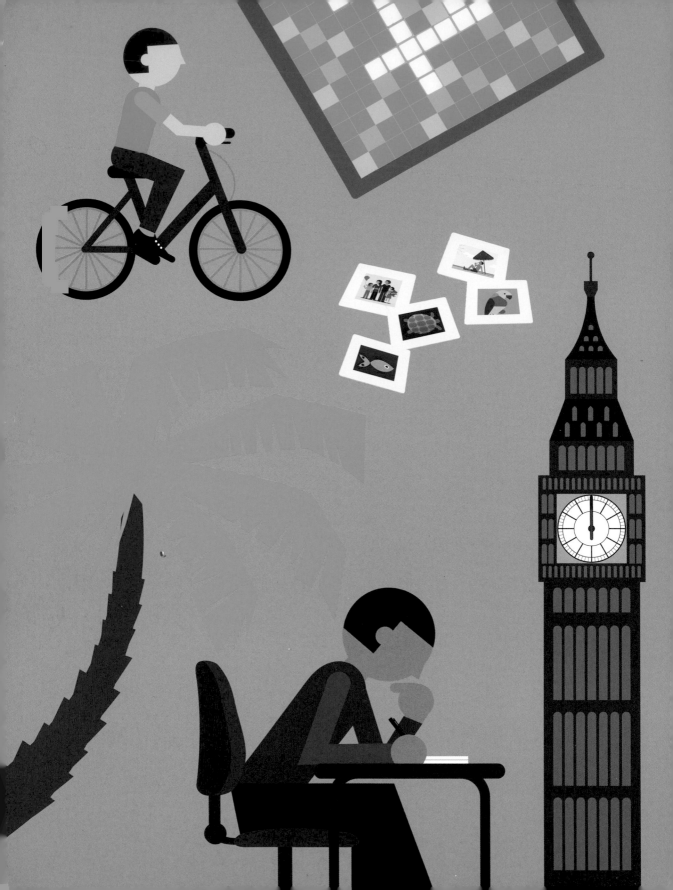

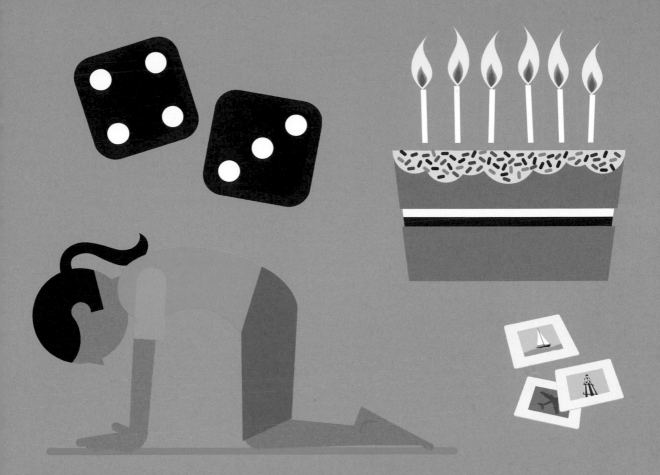

MAX YOUR MEMORY
the complete **visual** program

Dr. Pascale Michelon

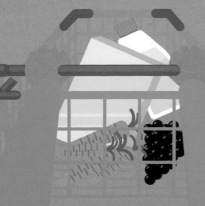

LONDON, NEW YORK, MUNICH,
MELBOURNE, AND DELHI

Illustrator Keith Hagan at
www.greenwich-design.co.uk
Project editor Suhel Ahmed
Project art editor Charlotte Seymour
Designer Nicola Erdpresser
Editor Angela Baynham
Assistant to illustrator Sarah Holland
Senior production editor Jennifer Murray
Production editor Marc Staples
US editor Jill Hamilton
Production controller Alice Holloway
Creative technical support Sonia Charbonnier
Managing editors Penny Warren and Penny Smith
Managing art editor Marianne Markham
Art director Peter Luff
Catergory publisher Peggy Vance

First American edition, 2012
Published in the United States by
DK Publishing, 375 Hudson Street
New York, NY 10014

12 13 14 15   10 9 8 7 6 5 4 3 2 1

001–182627–Jan/2012
Copyright © 2012
Dorling Kindersley Limited
All rights reserved.

Published in Great Britain by Dorling Kindersley Limited.

A CIP catalog record for this book is available from the
Library of Congress.

ISBN 978-0-7566-8965-0

Printed and bound in Singapore by Tien Wah Press

Discover more at
www.dk.com

DK books are available at special
discounts when purchased in
bulk for sales promotions,
premiums, fund-raising, or
educational use. For details,
contact: DK Publishing Special
Markets, 375 Hudson Street,
New York, New York 10014
or SpecialSales@dk.com.

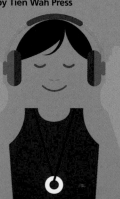

Contents

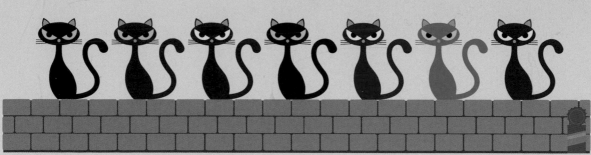

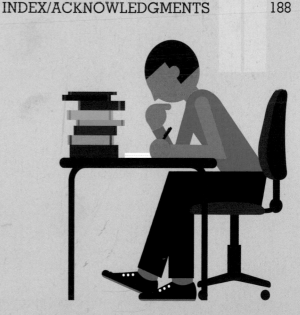

How to use this book

A visual program

If there is one magic word to open the door to a better memory, this word has to be "picture." It is a fact that pictures are easier to remember than words. As you will see, the method behind the majority of the memory-enhancing techniques presented in this book is to translate information into striking visual images and register these to enable better recall. This is one of the main reasons why *Max Your Memory* is a book that's visually led with fun and engaging illustrations and short chunks of easily digestible text.

Since learning becomes much easier when it is fun and relevant to us, most of the exercises throughout the book are not abstract but relate to familiar, everyday situations.

The chapters

The first step to boosting memory is to understand what memory is and how it works. Chapter 1 offers a clear, illustrated introduction to memory and brain potential. Chapters 2 and 3 focus on short-term and long-term memory respectively. The next two chapters offer key memory-enhancing techniques based on visualization and imagination (Chapter 4) and organization (Chapter 5). The book then explores memory for names (Chapter 6) and numbers (Chapter 7) and introduces key methods to improve memory capacity for both. The final chapter looks at some of the tweaks you can make to your lifestyle to maximize brain health: this includes information on nutrition, ways to manage stress, and tips to get adequate sleep and exercise.

"Super technique" pages offer proven methods for boosting memory power

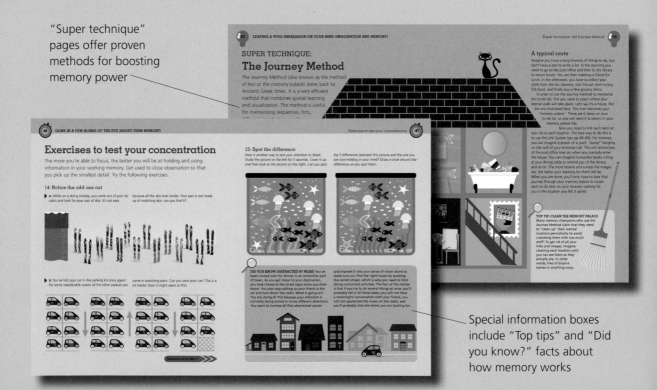

Special information boxes include "Top tips" and "Did you know?" facts about how memory works

Working through the book

The book is structured so that you can either choose a specific topic and focus on it alone, or work your way through from cover to cover. Chapters 2–7 start with check-in exercises to assess your current aptitude for a specific type of memory, e.g. long-term memory. Following a run-down of the key techniques and strategies, the check-out exercises at the end of the chapters encourage you to use these memory-boosting methods plus other tips to complete the exercises. You can then assess whether using these techniques has helped improve your memory.

Most of the exercises will ask you to memorize information and then cover it up, for which you will need a sheet of paper. In most instances, you will be asked to recall the information in the answer space provided. In cases where an answer space is not available, you will need an additional piece of paper to write down your answer. For exercises that test your long-term memory, you will be asked to complete an unrelated task to create a suitable time lag. These tasks will either be embedded in the question or framed in an illustrated tablet computer, which appears next to the main exercise.

Solutions

Finally, when applicable, you will find the solutions to the exercises at the back of the book. Look out for the solutions arrow on the relevant pages, which guides you to the specific page number.

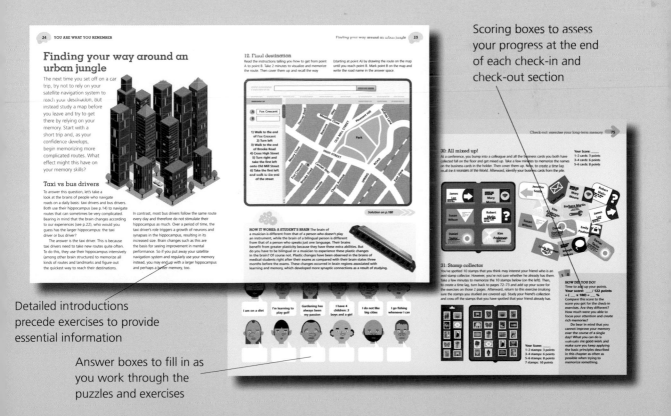

Scoring boxes to assess your progress at the end of each check-in and check-out section

Detailed introductions precede exercises to provide essential information

Answer boxes to fill in as you work through the puzzles and exercises

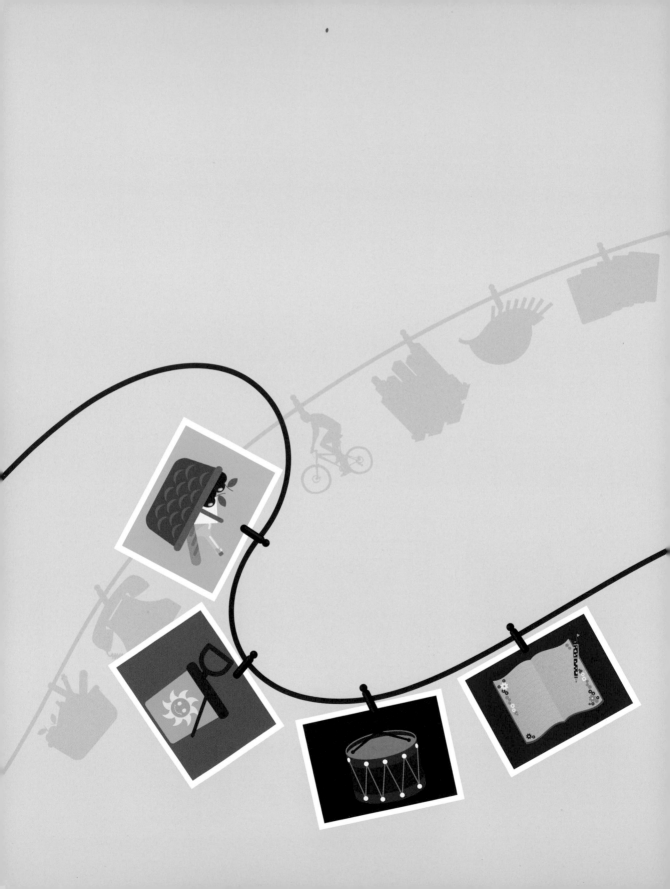

CHAPTER 1
YOU ARE WHAT YOU REMEMBER

What is memory?

Can you imagine living in the instant with no memories of the immediate or distant past? This is almost impossible to conceive—without any history or context, how would you know who the people talking to you are, what your favorite color is, and what to make of things happening around you?

Organizing memories

Memory allows us to store and retrieve information about the world and how we react to it, which is vital to understanding who we are, our relationships with the people around us, and what the world means to us. In order to understand how memory works, imagine filing away into a photo album a set of photographs from your trip last summer. First, you need to identify what each photograph refers to. Then you need to put the photos in the right chronological order in the album. You are doing this so that when you want

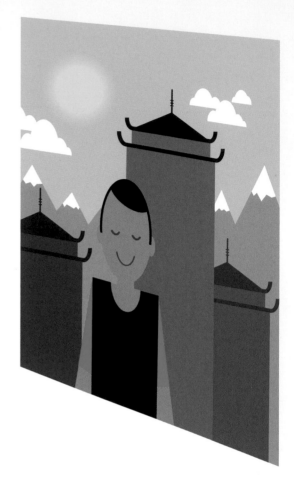

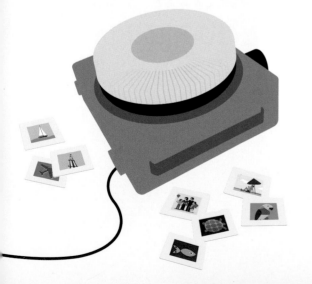

to recount any part of the experience again, you can refer back to the album and retrieve the right photo without a problem. These three actions, namely, registering (also called encoding), storing, and retrieving, are the three steps involved in memorization.

A solid memory forms when it has been well registered because it can then be retrieved easily. As you will find out throughout this book, there are many things you can do to improve your memory. You will learn techniques to enrich information with meaning so that you make information more memorable when you register it. This will provide you with cues to retrieve it later on.

1: Using your mind's eye

Let's look at what happens in the mind when you register information you read in a text. Read this short passage and visualize the scene.

"It was a beautiful day, perfect for a picnic. The air smelled fresh. Flowers could be seen all around the park. Julie found an ideal spot under a large tree to unfold her blanket and set up her basket. Since the tree had not completely bloomed yet, the sun was shining through and warming her legs. As she pulled out her food, she noticed the light shimmering on the water ahead of her."

Now answer the questions on the right referring to the details you visualized:

A: What was the time of year?

B: What color were the flowers?

C: What kind of tree did Julie settle under?

D: What color was Julie's blanket?

E: What types of food did Julie take out of her basket?

F: What kind of water feature caught Julie's attention?

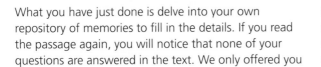

What you have just done is delve into your own repository of memories to fill in the details. If you read the passage again, you will notice that none of your questions are answered in the text. We only offered you cues to trigger your imagination, which tapped into the vast archive of information you already possess. The visual details you recall when reading a text are powerful cues that can help you retrieve what you read later on.

TOP TIP: CREATE VISUAL MEANING So how does your mind process information? The information is first analyzed and registered. For example, take the Spanish word "vaca" written above the picture of a cow. Your brain will identify the word and associate it with the visual image. So far so good: you know that you are reading the word "vaca" and that it means "cow" in Spanish. You have a good chance of remembering this, but your memory may be enhanced further if you also create visual meaning. How? Take a mental snapshot of the two pieces of information together. This way your brain will register the relationship between the object and the word. In doing so, you will increase the likelihood of remembering the word because visual information sticks in the mind more readily.

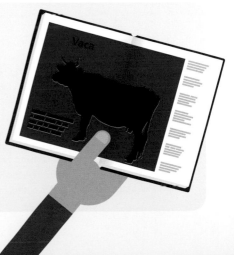

Is memory automatic?

Try out these two exercises to learn more about how memory works. You'll find out whether it is always necessary to make a concerted effort to memorize in order to allow recall of information, or whether some things are memorized automatically.

2: Day at the beach

You are at the beach. Count how many toys you can put away directly (those on the table and chair) and how many you will have to clean up first (those on the sand).

Now cover up the picture. Although you weren't asked to memorize any of the toys, can you remember details about them? Answer these 5 questions:

A: Was the rubber duck wearing a hat?

B: What color was the octopus?

C: What is the picture of on the bucket?

D: Were there any stars on the ball?

E: What color was the truck's dumpster?

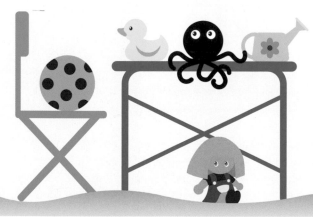

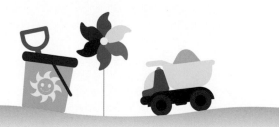

HOW IT WORKS: BRAIN ON AUTOPILOT So do you always consciously commit stuff to memory? Or do you sometimes remember things without even trying? After completing exercises 2 and 3, you probably found that you registered some information unconsciously! The brain registers many facts and details without you being aware of them. It makes sense when you think about it: life would become exhausting if you were always telling yourself to remember everything. Although most of the information we register automatically never becomes conscious, the brain constantly refers to it to build or reinforce our ideas about the world around us.

3: It's a matter of size

Would these commonly known objects fit in a regular shoebox? Write "yes" or "no" in the answer box provided for each object. Then cover up the objects.

Although you didn't memorize what the various objects were or how they were grouped together, can you remember which objects were placed on which table?

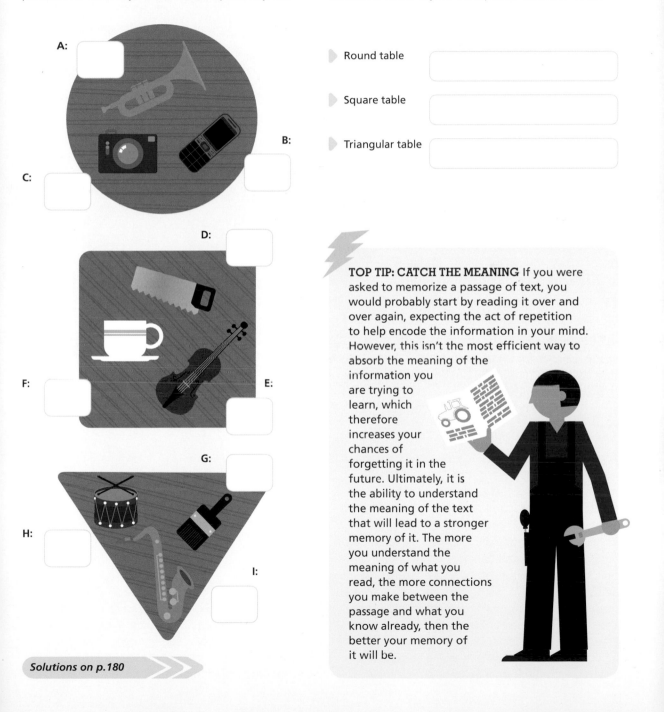

A:

B:

C:

D:

F:

E:

G:

H:

I:

Round table

Square table

Triangular table

TOP TIP: CATCH THE MEANING If you were asked to memorize a passage of text, you would probably start by reading it over and over again, expecting the act of repetition to help encode the information in your mind. However, this isn't the most efficient way to absorb the meaning of the information you are trying to learn, which therefore increases your chances of forgetting it in the future. Ultimately, it is the ability to understand the meaning of the text that will lead to a stronger memory of it. The more you understand the meaning of what you read, the more connections you make between the passage and what you know already, then the better your memory of it will be.

Solutions on p.180

Where in the brain do you keep your memories?

Are your memories stored at the back of your brain or at the front? Do we even know? Years of research have shown scientists that memories are not stored in any single place in the brain.

The main lobes

The brain weighs about 3 lb 5 oz (1.5 kg) and can be divided into two hemispheres, right and left. Each of these can in turn be divided into four major lobes: the occipital lobe (situated at the back of the head, above the neck), the temporal lobe (situated beside the temples), the frontal lobe (situated just behind the forehead), and the parietal lobe (situated in the back of the head, at the top). It turns out that each lobe within the brain is responsible for different skills and functions.

What the lobes do

The occipital lobe is devoted entirely to analyzing what we see. The parietal lobe is primarily responsible for attention, sensations such as touch, temperature, and pain, and spatial orientation. The frontal lobe is known for its role in higher abilities, which include decision-making, reasoning, impulse control, social behavior, and memory. The temporal lobe deals mostly with the senses of hearing and smell, as well as language and memory. Located deep inside the temporal lobe is the limbic system, and the different parts of this support our appetites, emotions, and instincts. One part in particular, the hippocampus, is critical for learning because it is involved with the formation of new memories.

A:

C:

B:

D:

As you can see, memory cannot be pinpointed to one specific part of the brain, but is dispersed throughout the different lobes and other sites. To summarize, a memory is the recollection and reconstruction of several pieces of information pulled together by mechanisms spread throughout the brain.

4: Label the brain

How much of what you have read so far can you remember? See if you can label this brain correctly by referring to the list on the right.

> Sections of the brain:
>
> Occipital lobe
> Temporal lobe
> Frontal lobe
> Parietal lobe
> Limbic system
> Hippocampus

E:

F:

Solutions on p.180 ⟫⟫

HOW IT WORKS: NIMBLE NEURONS When you remember the face of a loved one, it is the result of the activity of brain cells (or neurons) in specific parts of your brain. Active neurons transmit information to each other using electrical impulses as well as chemical molecules, called neurotransmitters. This exchange occurs very rapidly through synapses (the tiny gaps between neurons). An average brain contains roughly 100 billion neurons. What's more, each neuron is connected to approximately 10,000 other neurons. This goes some way toward explaining our limitless capacity for creating and storing memories.

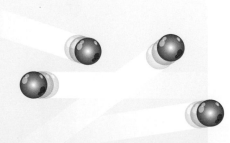

Why do we forget?

Our brain has the ability to hold on to lots of memories. However, it doesn't seem to keep hold of each one indefinitely. For example, you might never forget the name of your first love but always find it hard to remember where you left your keys. Why do we forget such things? As you know, memory works by first registering information and later retrieving it: things can go awry at either or both stages.

The science of forgetting

Let's look first at failure to register. Information that is registered poorly will be hard to retrieve. For example, it will be difficult to remember someone's name if you weren't paying enough attention when you were introduced to that person.

Now let's look at retrieval failures. One possibility is that memories just fade away over time, especially if they are no longer accessed. Another possibility is that memories interfere with each other. For instance, you may not remember where you parked your car today because of interference from memories of where you parked your car yesterday.

Finally, since most memories are attached to a context, a change of context may prevent you from retrieving a memory. For example, you might have trouble recalling the name of someone from your art class if you bump into that person in the supermarket. This would happen because the contextual cues usually associated with this person, namely, the classroom setting, the teacher, and the other students, are absent in the supermarket.

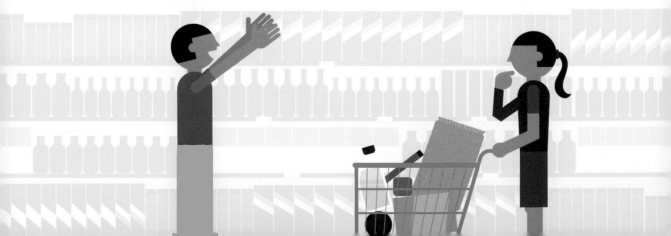

5: Reading to the beat

Read the passage below. At the same time, tap your middle and index fingers on the table every 4 counts (count silently in your head). Once you've finished reading, cover it up, and answer the questions:

A: What was the forgetful person's name?

B: Who asked him to go to the store?

C: What was he supposed to buy?

D: What did he have to come back home for?

E: What kind of meat did he end up buying?

F: How many books did he return to the library?

Joe was a forgetful person. He was always losing his keys and leaving his wallet at home. One day his mother asked him to run to the store and buy a pint of milk, some bread and a packet of sausages. He came back an hour later after realizing that he forgot to take any money with him. His second trip was more successful even though he forgot the milk and instead bought a roast chicken. In the afternoon he managed to return six of his overdue books to the library.

Was it difficult to answer these questions? Finger drumming while reading the text divided your attention, which probably lowered your ability to register the information. This is an example of registering failure.

DID YOU KNOW: TIMES WHEN YOU WANT TO FORGET Have you seen the Hollywood movie *Eternal Sunshine of the Spotless Mind*? In the film a couple undergo a procedure to erase each other from their memories when their relationship turns sour. We'd all like to forget some memories, especially those that are traumatic. To date, there is no such procedure as the one depicted in the movie. However, one way memories can be suppressed is by actively trying to exclude them from our conscious thoughts. Although this may sound paradoxical, the process of conscious suppression has been shown to work in psychological experiments. Another way memories might be suppressed is by an unconscious mechanism called repression.

Exercises to show why we forget

How about doing a few more exercises to understand the nature of memory recall and forgetfulness? To experience interference first hand, try exercise 6. To feel the power of emotions on memory, as well as the benefit of cues when attempting to recall the past, try exercises 7 and 8.

6: Mixing up the lists

Below is a grocery list. Can you memorize it in 1 minute? When you are done, hide the words.

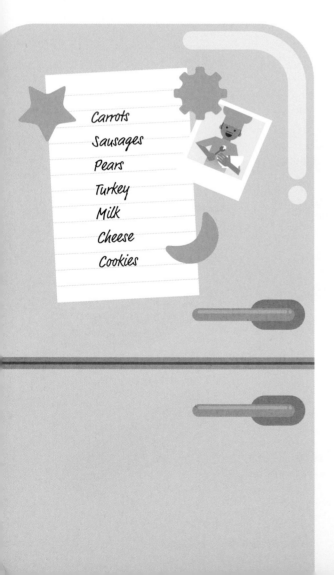

Carrots
Sausages
Pears
Turkey
Milk
Cheese
Cookies

Here are the words that your niece wrote in a spelling test. Can you check that they are all correctly spelled? Mark a check or an "x" beside each spelling.

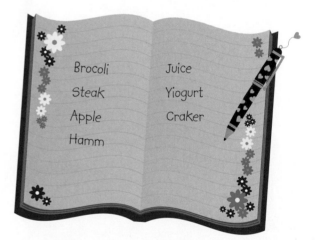

Brocoli   Juice
Steak   Yiogurt
Apple   Craker
Hamm

Do you still remember the grocery list you memorized? Try to write all the items down below.

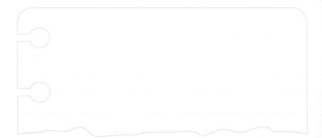

How did you find that? Did you incorrectly write down some of the words from your niece's spelling test? This is a perfect example of interference in memory: both lists contained food items and those got mixed up in your mind, causing you to commit retrieval errors.

7: I wish I could forget

Look at each picture for 1 second then hide them all.
Then try to write down as many pictures as you can recall.

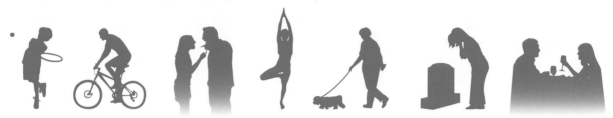

Did the two emotionally charged pictures feature in your answers? Unfortunately, negative or traumatic events tend to stick in our memory and are usually harder to forget. This is probably a way for us to catalog negative experiences in our brain so that we can hopefully protect ourselves from something similar happening in the future.

8: Wonderful cues

Take no more than 30 seconds to memorize the names of the 8 Ancient Wonders of the World listed below. Cover up the names, count aloud to 15, and then using the country names as cues to help recall, write down the name of each wonder in the box next to the country to which it belongs.

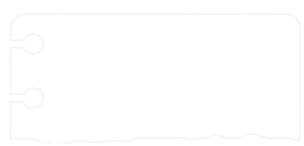

Peru	Machu Picchu
China	The Great Wall of China
Turkey	The Temple of Artemis
India	The Taj Mahal
Italy	The Leaning Tower of Pisa
Greece	The Statue of Zeus
Iraq	The Hanging Gardens of Babylon
Egypt	The Great Pyramid

China

Egypt

Iraq

Turkey

Peru

India

Italy

Greece

Can you improve your memory?

We are born with a finite memory capacity and nothing can be done about that. Would you say that this statement is true or false? Of course it's false! Your memory can be trained and improved at any age throughout your life.

Mnemonics

Great examples demonstrating the talents of a trained memory can be found in societies (past and present) that rely on the use of oral tradition in the absence of written language. In these cases, human memory is the only way to store knowledge. A few individuals have to become memory experts. They train their memories so that they can orally pass knowledge on to future generations.

Unfortunately, there is no easy pill you can take to boost memory. Your memory will get better only if you use it regularly. Your memory will also improve if you use mnemonics. A mnemonic is the name given to any technique that helps your memory store information. Mnemonics were used by the Ancient Greeks and they are still used today, especially by competitors at memory competitions around the world.

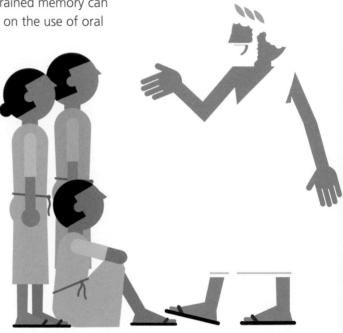

DID YOU KNOW: PRACTICE MAKES PERFECT Have you heard of Joshua Foer, the 2006 record holder in speed cards at the USA Memory Championships? In a "speed-card" contest, competitors race to memorize a pack of playing cards. Joshua Foer took only 1 minute and 40 seconds to memorize his pack successfully. A year earlier, Foer was a young journalist and a novice in the domain of memory training. He had decided to train to become a memory expert and it worked! How did he do that? He used mnemonics, especially those that involved creating complex visual images that would readily stick in his mind.

9: Memorize fun facts

How about starting your memory-improving course by trying to memorize these fun facts? You never know, they may come in handy if you're taking part in a quiz, or if you just want to impress friends.

Take 2 minutes to memorize these facts. Then cover them up and write down as many as you can remember. The pictures below should help. Later today, recount at least 2 of these facts to someone you know.

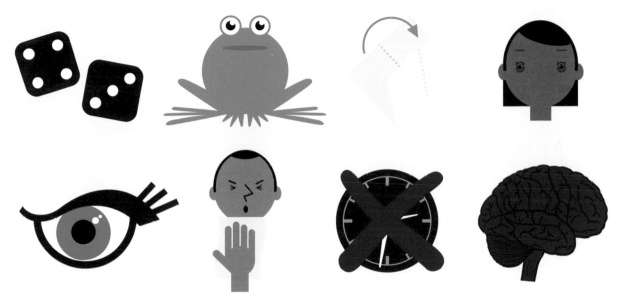

▷ **A:** The opposite sides of a die always add up to 7.

▷ **B:** Frogs never close their eyes, even when they are sleeping.

▷ **C:** No piece of paper can be folded more than 7 times.

▷ **D:** A human eye has 6 muscles that control its movements.

▷ **E:** The pupil is actually a hole in the center of the eye: it allows light to enter the retina.

▷ **F:** About 25 percent of human beings sneeze when they look up at a bright sky.

▷ **G:** There are no clocks in Las Vegas gambling casinos.

▷ **H:** We use 100 percent of our brain, not just 10 percent.

Your plastic brain

No, your brain is not made of plastic! It is not a muscle either. But your brain has the ability to change depending on your daily experiences. This ability is called "plasticity" or "neuroplasticity" to be precise.

Plastic changes

Changes in the brain occur at the level of the synapses (the connections between neurons, see p.15). Exposed to challenging tasks, the synapses eventually become more efficient. The experience of the task also causes new synaptic connections to appear. The same can be said about neurons, with new ones also appearing and growing, even in an adult brain. This occurs especially in the hippocampus (this region is crucial for memory formation, see p.14). As you can probably guess, changes in the brain do not happen in a single day, but over a long period of time through the repeated use of a specific part of the brain.

Plastic changes occur a lot during childhood as the brain grows and matures. These changes can also take place following a brain injury. For instance, with access to proper rehabilitation, a person who has suffered

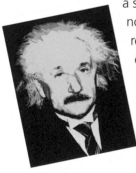

a stroke can recover the use of an apparently nonfunctional limb thanks to neuronal reorganization in the brain. Finally, plastic changes occur during adulthood whenever new things are learned, memorized, and rehearsed. The good news is that the more you learn and memorize, the more connections are created and strengthened in your brain, which helps boost your ability to register and retrieve information.

10: Wastebasket ball

Here is a simple exercise to demonstrate how repeated practice can lead to better performance. Your brain isn't likely to change dramatically during the course of this exercise, but it would if you were to challenge yourself by taking up a musical instrument, for example.

Use a wastebasket and a sheet of paper scrunched into a ball. Throw the "ball" repeatedly until you get 3 successful throws in a row. Increase the distance between you and the basket. Do the same exercise. With practice, you should find your aim improving over time.

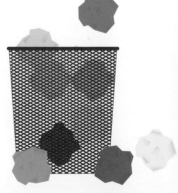

11: Useful phone numbers

How much do you try to memorize on a daily basis? Let's test your memory for phone numbers you probably use quite often. Mark an "x" in the answer space if you do not know the answer.

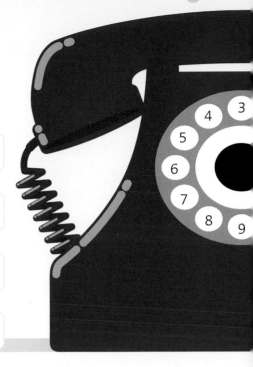

A: What is your closest friend's phone number?

B: What is your doctor's phone number?

C: What are the phone numbers of the two family members you call most often?

D: What is your dentist's phone number?

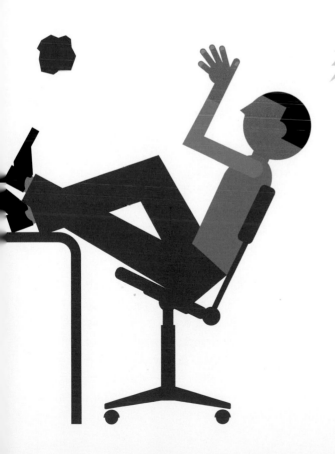

TOP TIP: USE YOUR MEMORY How well did you perform in the above exercise? If you couldn't answer any of the questions, then it's a good indication that you didn't memorize the numbers in the first place. There's nothing strange about that. In fact, why bother memorizing these numbers when your mobile phone, computer, or sticky notes can do it for you? Therein lies the problem. We tend to rely a lot on external aids these days and thus fail to use and develop our huge internal potential. One way to take advantage of neuroplasticity to boost memory is to use your memory on a daily basis. As you enter a number in your mobile phone, why not try to memorize it? You can do the same thing when you have only a few items to get from the store or when you write a date in your diary.

Throw me away!

Finding your way around an urban jungle

The next time you set off on a car trip, try not to rely on your satellite navigation system to reach your destination, but instead study a map before you leave and try to get there by relying on your memory. Start with a short trip and, as your confidence develops, begin memorizing more complicated routes. What effect might this have on your memory skills?

Taxi vs bus drivers

To answer this question, let's take a look at the brains of people who navigate roads on a daily basis: taxi drivers and bus drivers. Both use their hippocampus (see p.14) to navigate routes that can sometimes be very complicated. Bearing in mind that the brain changes according to our experiences (see p.22), who would you guess has the larger hippocampus: the taxi driver or bus driver?

The answer is the taxi driver. This is because taxi drivers need to take new routes quite often. To do this, they use their hippocampus intensively (among other brain structures) to memorize all kinds of routes and landmarks and figure out the quickest way to reach their destinations.

In contrast, most bus drivers follow the same route every day and therefore do not stimulate their hippocampus as much. Over a period of time, the taxi driver's role triggers a growth of neurons and synapses in the hippocampus, resulting in its increased size. Brain changes such as this are the basis for seeing improvement in mental performance. So if you put away your satellite navigation system and regularly use your memory instead, you may end up with a larger hippocampus and perhaps a better memory, too.

12: Final destination

Read the instructions telling you how to get from point A to point B. Take 2 minutes to visualize and memorize the route. Then cover them up and recall the way (starting at point A) by drawing the route on the map until you reach point B. Mark point B on the map and write the road name in the answer space.

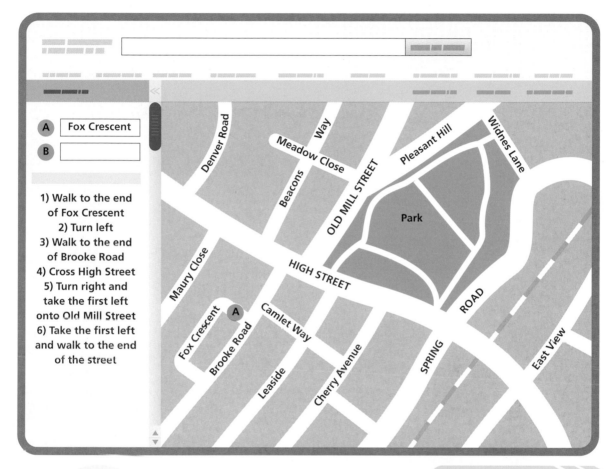

A   Fox Crescent

B

1) Walk to the end of Fox Crescent
2) Turn left
3) Walk to the end of Brooke Road
4) Cross High Street
5) Turn right and take the first left onto Old Mill Street
6) Take the first left and walk to the end of the street

Solution on p.180

HOW IT WORKS: A STUDENT'S BRAIN The brain of a musician is different from that of a person who doesn't play an instrument, while the brain of a bilingual person is different from that of a person who speaks just one language. Their brains benefit from greater plasticity because they have these extra abilities. But do you have to be bilingual or a musician to experience these plastic changes in the brain? Of course not. Plastic changes have been observed in the brains of medical students right after their exams as compared with their brain states three months before the exams. These changes occurred in brain regions associated with learning and memory, which developed more synaptic connections as a result of studying.

Check-out

How attentively have you been reading this chapter? How much of it can you recall? Answer the questions below to test your memory for what you have learned so far. As you will find out in chapter 3, testing your memory for what you have recently learned is one of the best ways to register new information.

13: The memory quiz

Circle the correct answer for each question. Do not refer back to the chapter to search for any of the answers, but try to rely on your memory alone.

1. Memories are located in a specific place in the brain.
A: True
B: False
C: Depends on the individual

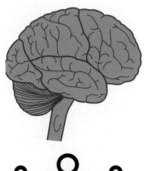

2. Mnemonics have been around since:
A: Ancient Greek times
B: the 12th century
C: the 18th century

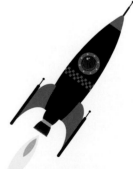

3. An average brain weighs approximately:
A: 3 lb 5 oz (1.5 kg)
B: 5 lb (2.3 kg)
C: 4 lb (1.8 kg)

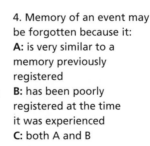

4. Memory of an event may be forgotten because it:
A: is very similar to a memory previously registered
B: has been poorly registered at the time it was experienced
C: both A and B

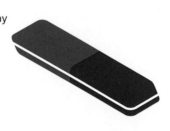

5. What is the name of the lobe behind your forehead?
A: The parietal lobe
B: The occipital lobe
C: The frontal lobe

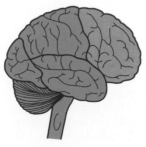

6. When registering information you can boost your memory by:
A: forming visual images
B: drumming your fingers on the table
C: counting in your head

7. Information is memorized only when we make an effort to remember it.
A: True
B: False
C: Depends on age

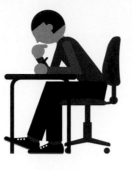
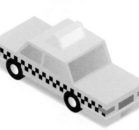

8. An average brain contains approximately:
A: 100 million neurons
B: 100 billion neurons
C: 100,000 neurons

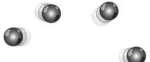

9. Taxi drivers have a larger hippocampus than bus drivers because:
A: taxi drivers need to take new routes quite often
B: taxi drivers drive a more complex vehicle
C: taxi drivers converse more with their passengers

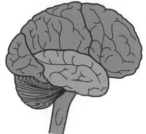

10. To say that the brain is plastic means that:
A: the brain is not mature when we are born
B: the brain changes according to our experiences
C: the brain's connections are fixed in adulthood

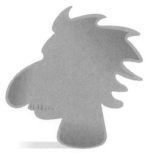

11. Which structure in the temporal lobe is important for memory formation?
A: The cerebellum
B: The hippocampus
C: The hypothalamus

12. Memory can be improved:
A: only until the age of 20
B: until middle age
C: throughout life

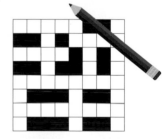

13. The different steps involved in memorization are:
A: register—store— retrieve
B: record—order— recall
C: register—imagine— recognize

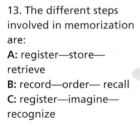
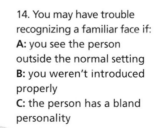

14. You may have trouble recognizing a familiar face if:
A: you see the person outside the normal setting
B: you weren't introduced properly
C: the person has a bland personality

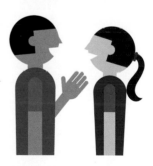

1   0

HOW DID YOU DO?
Time to add up your points. **Your score:**
_____ ÷ **14 points = (** _____ **x 100) =** _____ **%**
At the end of chapters 2–7, you will be tested with a set of check-out exercises. Compare this score with the check-in score at the start of each chapter to assess your overall progress.

Solutions on p.180

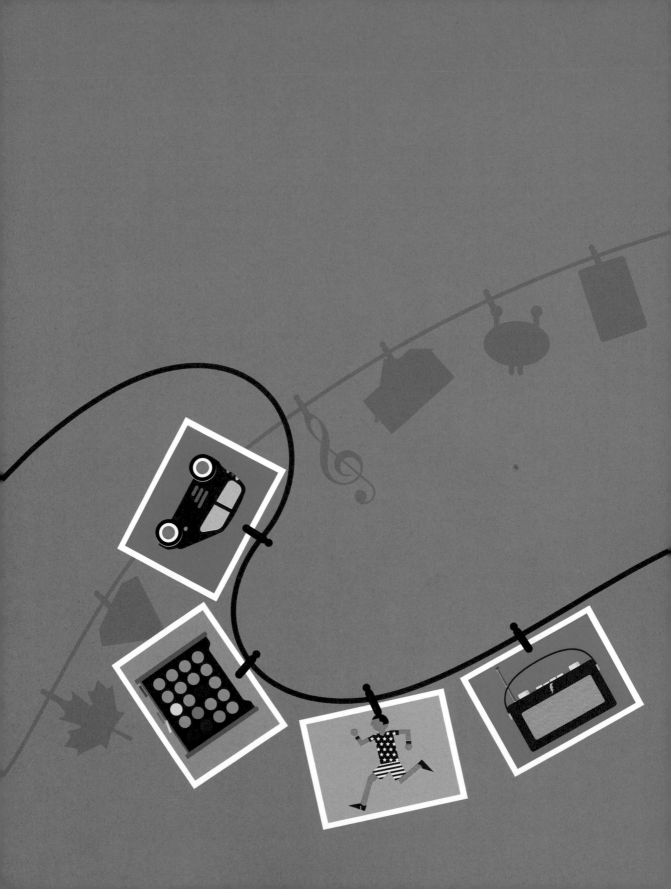

CHAPTER 2
GONE IN A FEW BLINKS OF THE EYE (SHORT-TERM MEMORY)

Check-in: how well do you remember the very recent past?

Memory for the very recent past (up to a minute ago) and memory for the past (everything beyond a minute) are different. The former is called short-term memory and the latter is known as long-term memory. Short-term memory allows you to hold in your mind what you have just heard, read, or seen. In the following exercises, your aim is to look at the material once, try to hold it in your mind, and then recall it as accurately as possible.

1: What is your limit?

Below are several series of numbers. To determine your memory span, starting with the shortest series, read the numbers once in your head and then cover up the series. Recall the numbers in the order you read them.

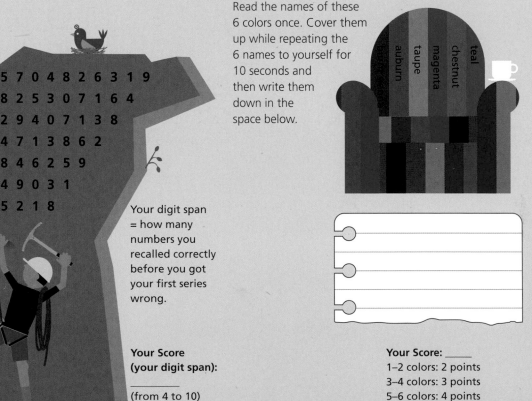

5 7 0 4 8 2 6 3 1 9

8 2 5 3 0 7 1 6 4

2 9 4 0 7 1 3 8

4 7 1 3 8 6 2

8 4 6 2 5 9

4 9 0 3 1

5 2 1 8

Your digit span = how many numbers you recalled correctly before you got your first series wrong.

Your Score (your digit span):

_____

(from 4 to 10)

2: Sofa colors

In a phone conversation, the salesperson at the furniture store tells you the 6 available colors for the armchair you want to buy. You need to remember the names of these colors until you can write them down on a piece of paper.

Read the names of these 6 colors once. Cover them up while repeating the 6 names to yourself for 10 seconds and then write them down in the space below.

auburn
taupe
magenta
chestnut
teal

Your Score: _____
1–2 colors: 2 points
3–4 colors: 3 points
5–6 colors: 4 points

3: Cluster of shapes

Study this picture of overlapping shapes for 5 seconds. Then cover it up and reproduce what you remember in the space provided.

Your Score: _____
2 errors+: 1 point
1–2 errors: 2 points
no errors: 3 points

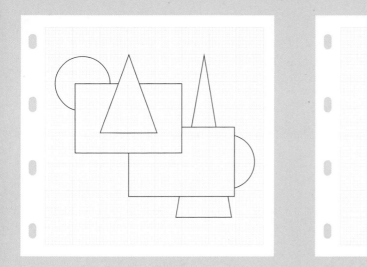

4: Cat invasion!

The 7 cats on the top wall have invaded your backyard. Look at them once, then cover them up and study the cats on the bottom wall. Very quickly, circle the cats that have never been in your backyard.

Your Score: _____
1 cat spotted: 1 point
2 cats: 2 points
3 cats: 3 points

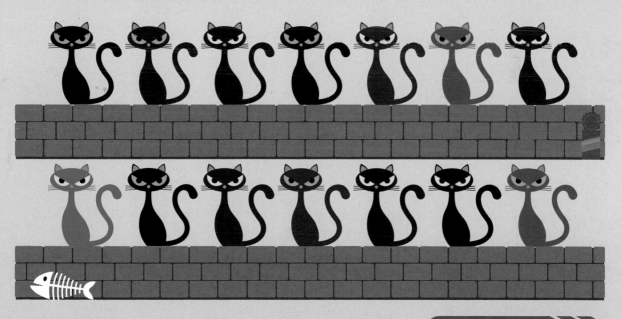

Solution on p.180

5: Write on your mental screen

You call for the check after a meal with friends at a restaurant and have to divide it up among the group. It's a situation familiar to most of us, and often we reach for the calculator feature on our phones rather than relying on mental arithmetic. Practice dividing these numbers in your head and see how many you get right.

Divide 120 by 3 =

Divide 125 by 5 =

Divide 46 by 2 =

Divide 96 by 6 =

Divide 300 by 12 =

Divide 140 by 4 =

Your Score: _____
1–2 correct: 2 points
3–4 correct: 3 points
5–6 correct: 4 points

Solutions on p.180

6: Gym locker

The receptionist at the gym gives you a new security code to access your locker. While rifling through your pockets for something to write it on, you have to hold the digits in your head for a few seconds. Read this series of digits once, then cover it up, and after 10 seconds write it in the space provided.

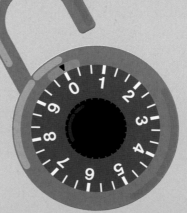

Your Score: _____
1–3 digits: 2 points
4–5 digits: 3 points
6–8 digits: 4 points

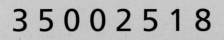

3 5 0 0 2 5 1 8

7: March of the animals

Quickly study this procession of animals. Pay attention to which animals are shown as well as their order (from left to right). Then cover them up. Imagine that all the animals have turned around and are heading back to where they came from. Can you list them all starting with the last one in the procession (i.e. the one on the right)?

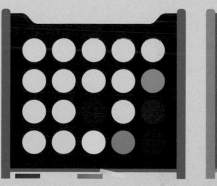

Your Score: _____
1–2 animals in the right place: 2 points
3–4 animals: 3 points
5–6 animals: 4 points

8: Four in a row

You are playing a popular game that involves arranging counters on a board. Unfortunately, during one game you accidentally knock the board over, so you have to recreate the arrangement from memory. Study the left board for 5 seconds. Then cover it up and reproduce the arrangement in the board on the right (you can either write the initial of the correct color in the appropriate circle, or color it in).

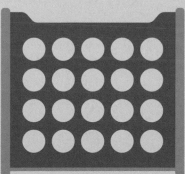

Your Score: _____
1–2 counters: 2 points
3–4 counters: 3 points
5–6 counters: 4 points

HOW DID YOU DO?
Time to add up your points.
Your score: _____ ÷ 36 points
= (_____ x 100) = _____ %
Are you surprised by your performance? Did you do better than you thought you would? In the next pages, you'll read about how your short-term memory helps you keep in mind a wide range of information, from a phone number while you are dialing it, to the shade of a color while you are painting. As you will discover, focus is key to improving your short-term memory.

What is short-term memory?

Your short-term memory allows you to hold a piece of information in your mind while you are performing a task. The information will fade rapidly unless you actively try to retain it. This is crucial so that information relevant to the next task can then be kept in mind.

Visual and verbal components

Depending on what you are holding in your mind, you use either your verbal or your visual short-term memory. If you are trying to remember a phone number someone just told you, you repeat it to yourself until you can write it down, thereby using your verbal, or "phonological," short-term memory. If you want to copy down something you briefly saw on a screen, you keep a picture of it in your head, using your visual short-term memory. Do the following exercises to test both components.

9: Where was it?

Take a look at this treasure map for no longer than 5 seconds and memorize the location of the hidden jewels. Then cover it up. Now mark on the empty grid below where the jewels were placed.

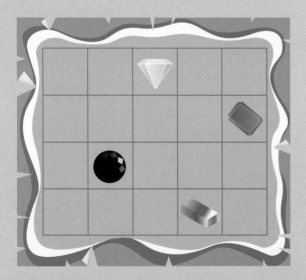

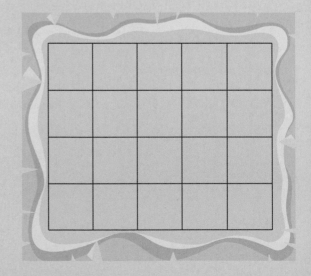

10: When order matters

Read each sequence of letters once, cover it up, and fill in the blanks.

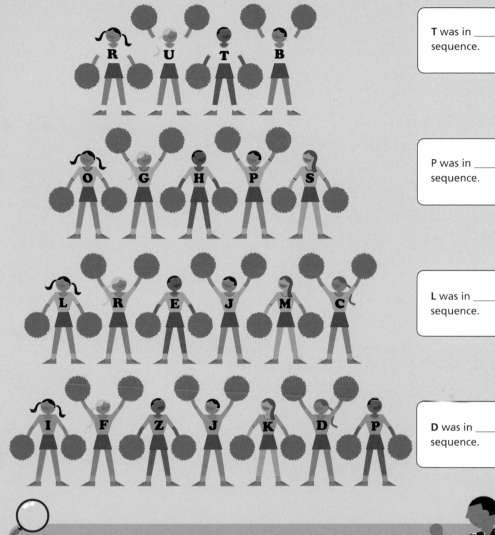

T was in _____ position in the sequence.

P was in _____ position in the sequence.

L was in _____ position in the sequence.

D was in _____ position in the sequence.

DID YOU KNOW: STUCK ON SEVEN Short-term memory capacity is limited. In the 1950s, a psychologist called George Miller identified the magic number 7: it is the number of items that most people can hold in their short-term memory (plus or minus 2). Not very impressive when you realize that most phone numbers are generally 10 digits long! In the 1980s, an American college student who wasn't a memory expert memorized over 70 digits that were read to him one after the other. How was that possible? Aside from lots of practice, he used a technique called chunking (see p.154). This is something you can do, too.

Visual short-term memory

Visual short-term memory (VSTM) helps us keep in mind visual and spatial information for a very limited period of time so that it can be used to carry out ongoing cognitive tasks. The information might include the shapes and colors of things as well as their location around us.

Our mental sketchpad

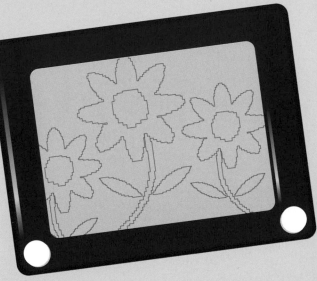

Did you know that while we're moving our eyes (which happens quite often), we are unable to see? It is during this process that the VSTM plays an important role: it helps automatically fill in the tiny gaps between eye movements by momentarily storing what the world looks like.

On a more conscious level, VSTM can be thought of as a mental sketchpad on which you constantly draw and erase information.

You use it when you compare objects that are not near each other, such as when you are trying to choose between two types of wallpaper that happen to be located in different aisles of the home design store. You use it when you're trying to parallel park your car by flitting your glance between the mirrors as you reverse into the tight space so as not to hit anything. You also rely on VSTM when you do spot-the-difference exercises. In all these cases, VSTM helps you retain visual information that is essential to complete the task at hand.

Using the mental sketchpad

Imagine a bowl of vanilla ice cream with a cherry on top. What you have just done is use your VSTM! All the images that appear in your mind's eye are formed on your mental sketchpad. You can then manipulate the image if that's what you need to do. (This process is discussed in detail on page 38.)

As you will find out throughout this book, the ability to visualize is important for boosting memory performance in general. This is a great motivation for stimulating your VSTM ability. You can begin right now by attempting the exercise on the next page.

11: Follow the path

Hold a path in your short-term memory. For each grid, briefly focus on the direction of the path and then cover it up. Hold the path in your mind's eye while counting to 5. Then reproduce the path in the empty grid.

TOP TIP: MINIMIZE DISTRACTIONS Both verbal and visual short-term memories are very susceptible to distraction. Any interruption while you are holding information in this manner can make it disappear. Completing complex tasks in an environment free of distractions is essential for success. Turning the radio off, muting your email alerts, and avoiding a screen saver that has a moving object are examples of simple things you can do to minimize distractions and help boost your short-term memory performance.

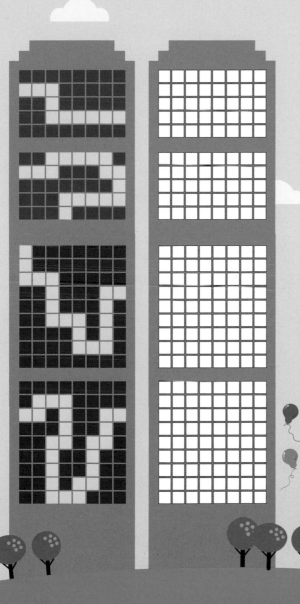

Working memory

Draw the letter J on your mental sketchpad. Now draw the letter D. Turn it 90° to the left and put it on top of the J. What does this shape resemble? An umbrella, of course! You've just used your working memory. Our working memory is a crucial part of the memory system, not least because it helps us to figure things out mentally.

Temporary workspace

Not only can we store information in our short-term memory, but we can also manipulate it. This is why short-term memory is sometimes also called the working memory. Working memory is our temporary workspace. We use it in everyday tasks ranging from driving (where you need to keep in mind the location of the cars around you as you navigate through traffic), to preparing a budget (where you need to keep in mind one spending category while working on another), to writing a letter (where you need to keep in mind all you want to say while developing each point a sentence at a time).

Active thinking

Increasing or maintaining one's working memory ability has enormous benefits in life. It could be compared to boosting the processing capacity of a computer. Working memory is where you do your active thinking and problem solving. So, a well-functioning working memory is key to successfully completing many complex activities that require you to reason, understand, and learn. Try the exercises opposite to use your mental workspace in different situations.

12: Mental rotation

When trying to find the right jigsaw puzzle piece, you often mentally rotate the ones you see on the table to "see" in your working mental space whether they would fit. Let's practice mental rotation here. In each box below, study each part of the top figure for 5 seconds. Then cover it up and circle the figure in the bottom part that matches it. You will have to mentally rotate the figures to find the answer.

13: Backward spelling

You are compiling a school quiz and one of the questions involves spelling several words backward. Before asking the pupils to take part, you decide to try it yourself. Work on one word at a time. Read the word once, then cover it up and spell it backward.

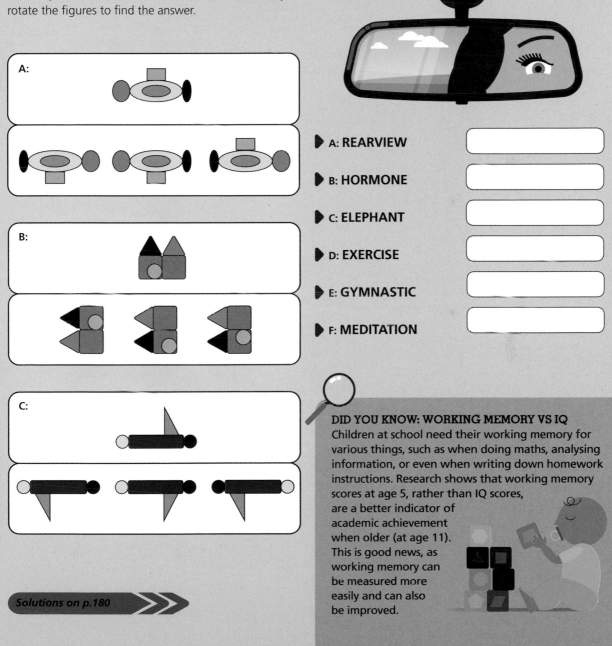

A: ▶ **A: REARVIEW**

▶ **B: HORMONE**

▶ **C: ELEPHANT**

▶ **D: EXERCISE**

B: ▶ **E: GYMNASTIC**

▶ **F: MEDITATION**

C:

DID YOU KNOW: WORKING MEMORY VS IQ
Children at school need their working memory for various things, such as when doing maths, analysing information, or even when writing down homework instructions. Research shows that working memory scores at age 5, rather than IQ scores, are a better indicator of academic achievement when older (at age 11). This is good news, as working memory can be measured more easily and can also be improved.

Solutions on p.180

SUPER TECHNIQUE:

Be attentive to boost your working memory

Imagine holding a set of directions in your memory while driving. If a billboard advertisement catches your attention, it may invade your mental workspace and cause you to forget these directions. The same thing may happen if an unrelated thought suddenly comes to mind. Information in working memory fades away unless it is refreshed. Maintaining information in your short-term memory requires a lot of attention. The more you are able to focus on task-relevant information and ignore distractions, the better your memory performance will be. Irrelevant thoughts that enter your mental workspace and divide your focus may lead to information overload and ultimately errors.

Does multitasking really work?

Most of us lead busy lives these days, and one of the ways in which we try to get everything done is through multitasking. Multitasking requires you to hold information relevant to two or more tasks simultaneously in your working memory. This happens, for example, when you try to talk on the phone while also you're calculating how much you've spent on your last shopping spree: you have to be mindful of what your conversation is about while entering numbers in your calculator. First of all, attending to two actvities at the same time means that you're forced to divide your attention, which allocates less attention power to each activity. Secondly, it is hard to store and manipulate a lot of information in this limited mental workspace. This is why multitasking often leads to errors, as opposed to greater efficiency. The basic principles relevant to boosting your working memory are listed in the box below.

Key memory-boosting principles

- Focus your attention on the task at hand.
- Reduce external distractions as much as possible.
- Avoid multitasking.
- Practice using your working memory—as with any brain function, working memory can become more efficient with practice.

HOW IT WORKS: WORKING MEMORY AND ADHD Increasing numbers of children seem to be diagnosed with Attention Deficit and Hyperactivity Disorder (ADHD). Although many parents seek medical help for this, is medication the best solution? Maybe not. ADHD usually goes hand in hand with working memory problems. Research has shown that training working memory leads to increased ability to focus attention and control impulses, and improved learning abilities. You can train working memory by performing regular computerized exercises that test powers of concentration.

Exercises to test your concentration

The more you're able to focus, the better you will be at holding and using information in your working memory. Get used to close observation so that you pick up the smallest detail. Try the following exercises.

14: Notice the odd one out

▶ **A:** While on a skiing holiday, you come out of your ski cabin and look for your pair of skis: it's not easy because all the skis look similar. Your pair is not made up of matching skis: can you find it?

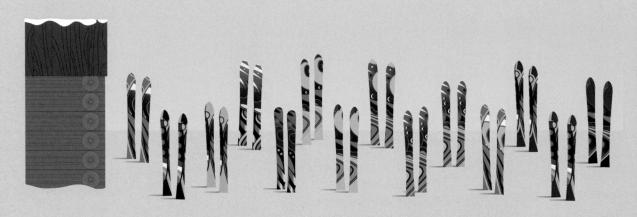

▶ **B:** You've lost your car in the parking lot once again! For some inexplicable reason all the other parked cars come in matching pairs. Can you spot your car? This is a lot harder than it might seem at first.

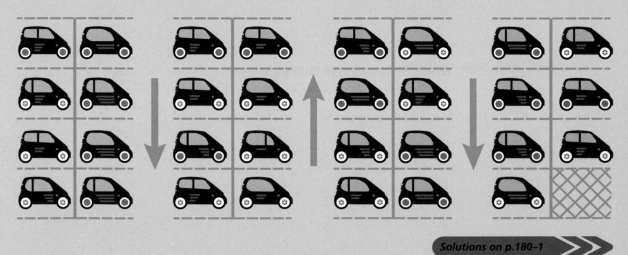

Solutions on p.180–1 ⟫⟫

15: Spot the difference

Here is another way to test your attention to detail. Study the picture on the left for 5 seconds. Cover it up and then look at the picture on the right. Can you spot the 5 differences between this picture and the one you are now holding in your mind? Draw a circle around the differences as you spot them.

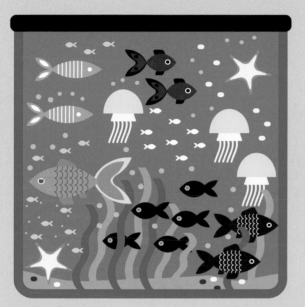

DID YOU KNOW: DISTRACTED BY NOISE You've been invited over for dinner in an unfamiliar part of town. As you get closer to your destination, you look closely at the street signs while you slow down. You also stop talking to your friend in the car and turn down the radio. What is going on? You are doing all this because your attention is currently being pulled in three different directions. You want to harness all that attentional power and channel it into your sense of vision alone to make sure you find the right house by spotting the correct street, which is why you need to limit doing concurrent activities. The fact of the matter is that if you try to do several things at once, you'll probably fail in all these tasks: you will not have a meaningful conversation with your friend, you will not appreciate the music on the radio, and you'll probably miss the street you are looking for.

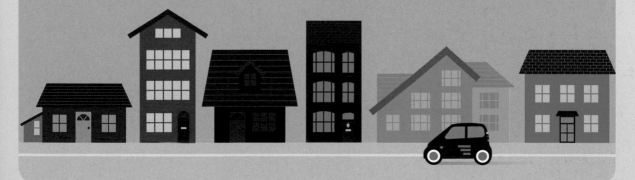

Check-out: exercise your short-term memory

Now that you know more about how your short-term memory and its various features work, as well as what you can do to try to boost it, let's assess how well you perform in the following exercises. Calculate your points for each exercise. Remember that attention is key here: eliminate potential distractions and make sure you maintain your focus throughout.

16: Letter strings

How many random letters can you hold in your mind? In other words, what's your letter span? Below are 7 series of letters. For each series, read the letters once in your head and then cover up the series. Recall the letters in the order you read them.

FTHU
UOSDB
NCRPAL
SIQMZTA
ONXIGUVR
EKDSPWACJ
HULDMQVAPI

17: Mixed-up numbers

The numbers for the price tags for your garage sale are on the table in a messy pile. You look at them while crossing the room and then wonder which numbers you have. To answer this question, take 5 seconds to study the image of the numbers below. Then cover them up and list the numbers you remember by referring to the picture in your head.

Your Score (your letter span):
_____ (from 4 to 10 points)

Your Score: _____
more than 2 errors: 1 point

1–2 errors: 2 points
no errors: 4 points

18: Team colors

You're off to watch a 5-a-side soccer tournament involving 5 teams. Below is information on the strip colors of the teams. Focus on one team at a time.

Read the different colors of each strip while trying to picture it on your mental screen. Then cover up the information and fill in the missing colors of each strip.

▶ **Team A:** RAPID ROVERS Red jersey, black shorts, blue socks with yellow trim, white boots

▶ **Team B:** STRIKE FORCE Green jersey with black collar, orange shorts, white socks, black boots

▶ **Team C:** DASHING DYNAMOS Blue jersey, white shorts, green socks with yellow trim, red boots

▶ **Team D:** SILKY TOUCH Yellow jersey with black collar, gray shorts, red socks with blue trim, white boots

▶ **Team E:** GOALS GALORE Black jersey, red shorts with white stripes, blue socks with yellow trim, red boots

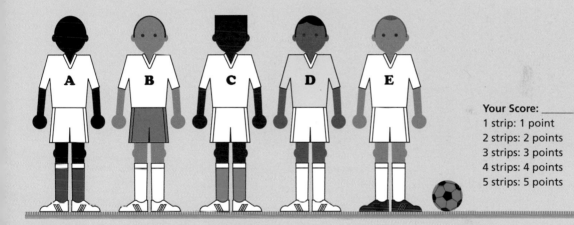

Your Score: _____
1 strip: 1 point
2 strips: 2 points
3 strips: 3 points
4 strips: 4 points
5 strips: 5 points

19: Jumbo sandwich

Your friend asks you to buy him a sandwich at lunchtime. You need to remember his order until you can write it down on a piece of paper. Read the names of these 7 ingredients once, cover them up, close your eyes for approximately 10 seconds while repeating the 7 ingredients to yourself, and then write them down in the answer space.

Ingredients: Swiss cheese, chicken, tomatoes, bacon, green peppers, lettuce, low-fat mayonnaise

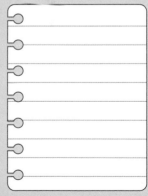

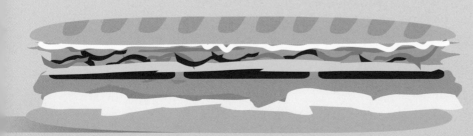

Your Score: _____
1–3 ingredients: 1 point
4–6 ingredients: 2 points
all ingredients: 4 points

20: Number position

Read each sequence of numbers once, cover it up, and fill in the blanks.

Your Score: _____
1 correct: 1 point
2 correct: 2 points
3 correct: 3 points
4 correct: 4 points

▶ **A:**

8 4 3 2 6 7

3 was in _____ position in the sequence

▶ **B:**

9 2 8 1 7 3 6 5

1 was in _____ position in the sequence

▶ **C:**

6 1 4 0 8 5 3 7

5 was in _____ position in the sequence

▶ **D:**

3 5 0 2 7 4 1 7 6 8

6 was in _____ position in the sequence

21: Put the items back

You accidentally bumped into the shelving unit and 5 items fell on the floor. Can you put them back where they were? Take 5 seconds to look at where each item is in the unit on the left. Then cover it up and draw arrows to show where the items on the floor should go in the unit on the right.

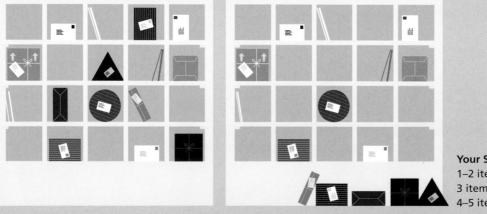

Your Score: _____
1–2 items: 2 points
3 items: 3 points
4–5 items: 4 points

22: Mental drawing

Let's test how accurately you can draw on your mental sketchpad. Using the instructions, make a mental drawing of the picture. Then cover up the instructions and draw what you have visualized in the space below.

A:
1. Visualize a large circle
2. Then a horizontal line dividing the circle in half
3. Then a vertical line dividing the circle in half
4. Then a square in the top left portion of the circle
5. Finally a triangle in the bottom right portion of the circle
Your drawing looks like this:

B:
1. Visualize a vertical line
2. Then a horizontal line crossing the vertical line through the middle
3. Then a circle attached to the top of the vertical line
4. Then a triangle attached to the right end of the horizontal line
5. Finally a rectangle attached to the bottom of the vertical line
Your drawing looks like this:

Your Score: _____
1 correct drawing: 2 points
2 correct drawings: 4 points

Solutions on p181

23: Alien visit

These 7 aliens appeared in your street. Look at each of them once. Cover them up and then look at the aliens on the right. Circle the aliens that did NOT appear in your street.

Your Score: _____ 1 alien spotted: 1 point
2 aliens: 2 points
3 aliens: 3 points

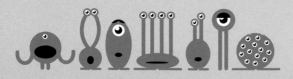
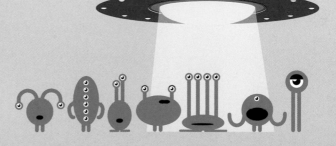

24: An orderly hand

For each set of playing cards, look at each card once while placing it on your mental screen. Then cover up the set and mentally reorder the cards beginning with the lowest value. Write down the name of the cards (including the suit they belong to) in their new order.

25: A day at the zoo

You want to create a memorable day for your family so have decided to take them to the zoo. At the entrance you see a map showing you where all the enclosures are located. Quickly look at the map below and then cover it up. Try to remember where the different animal enclosures are and fill in the empty map with the names of the animals

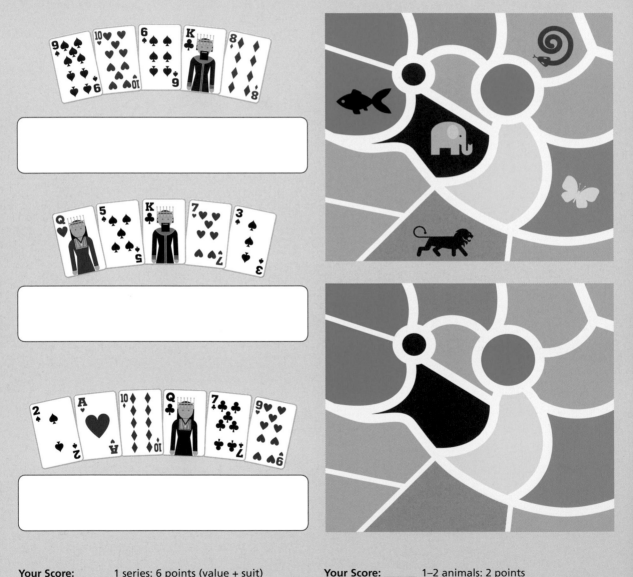

Your Score: _____ 1 series: 6 points (value + suit)
2 series: 8 points (value + suit)
3 series: 10 points (value + suit)

Your Score: _____ 1–2 animals: 2 points
3–4 animals: 3 points
5 animals: 4 points

26: Alien words

On the right is a list of words that were transmitted during an alien broadcast. Read each word once, then cover it up and spell it backward in the space below.

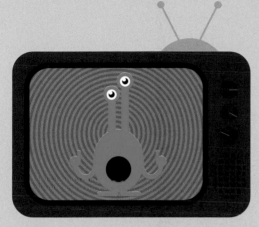

PRIGAL   ZATHERT

LUKAST

UFLITOR

SUVOLLEF

DEBOMET   *GRAXUM*

Your Score: _____   1–2 words spelled correctly: 2 points
3–4 words: 4 points
5–6 words: 6 points
7 words: 8 points

27: Can you sing backward?

▶ **A:** Do you know the lyrics of the nursery rhyme "Row row row your boat." Can you sing it backward? Think about each line and then sing or say it backward. Count how many lines you recite correctly in 1 minute.

▶ **B:** Now let's make it harder. Recite backward each line of the nursery rhyme "Humpty Dumpty." Once again you have 1 minute to recite as many lines as you can.

A: Your Score: _____ 1 line: 1 point
2 lines: 2 points
3–4 lines: 3 points

B: Your Score: _____
1 line: 1 point
2 lines: 2 points
3+ lines: 3 points

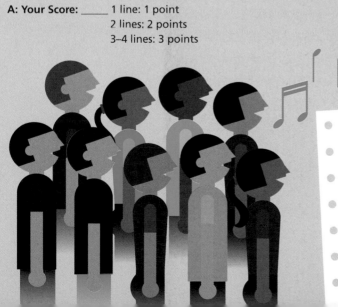

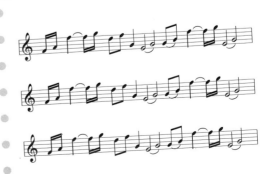

28: Finding your way

You are visiting a friend in an unfamiliar town. You ask a stranger for directions and she tells you how to get to your destination. Read the set of directions once. Then cover it up and, starting at point A in the map below, use your memory to draw the route to your destination. Let's see how many instructions you can remember.

1: Head westward and take the 1st right onto Easy Street
2: Keep walking northbound and take the 3rd left onto Bidas Walk
3: Walk to the end of Bidas Walk and turn right onto Judges Walk
4: Take the 1st left onto Chester Avenue and head to the end of the street

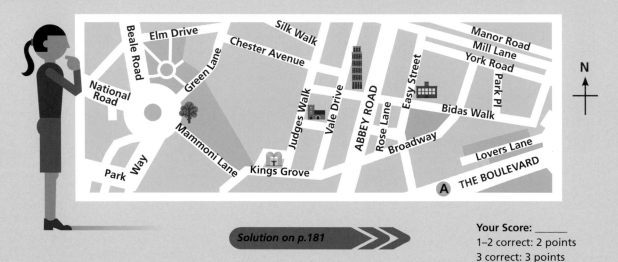

Solution on p.181

Your Score: _____
1–2 correct: 2 points
3 correct: 3 points
4 correct: 4 points

29: Gift time!

Can you mentally order these gifts starting with the smallest? Once you have done so, cover them up. Now refer to this new order and write down the color(s) of the 1st gift, the 2nd, and so on.

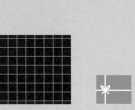
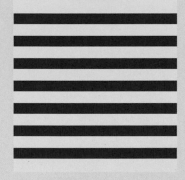
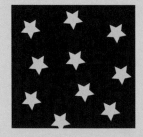
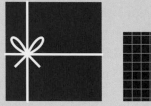

Your Score: _____
1–2 correct: 2 points
3–4 correct: 3 points
5 correct: 4 points

30: The flag game

Study the top 2 flag garlands for 5 seconds. Then cover them up and color in the blank spaces of the flags below, and write the name of the country each flag represents.

Your Score: _____
1–3 correct: 2 points
4–5 correct: 3 points
6–7 correct: 4 points
8+ correct: 5 points

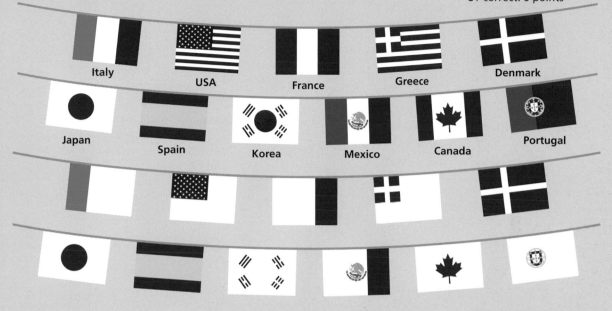

Italy   USA   France   Greece   Denmark

Japan   Spain   Korea   Mexico   Canada   Portugal

31: Identical layout

You have moved to a new house and want to arrange the furniture the way it was in your previous home. For each room, look at the objects and their location once. Then cover it up and draw them in the empty plan below.

Your Score: _____
1 room correct: 2 points
both rooms correct: 4 points

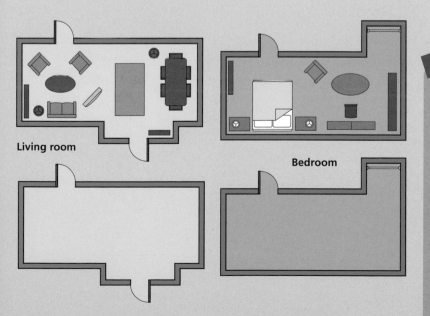

Living room

Bedroom

HOW DID YOU DO?
Time to add up your points.
Your score: _____ ÷ **83 points** = (_____ x 100) = _____ %
Compare this score to the score you got for the check-in exercises. Have you made any progress? Of course, your brain workout doesn't stop here. To expand your short-term and working memory capacity, make sure you use it regularly and, above all, don't forget that it's all about maintaining focus!

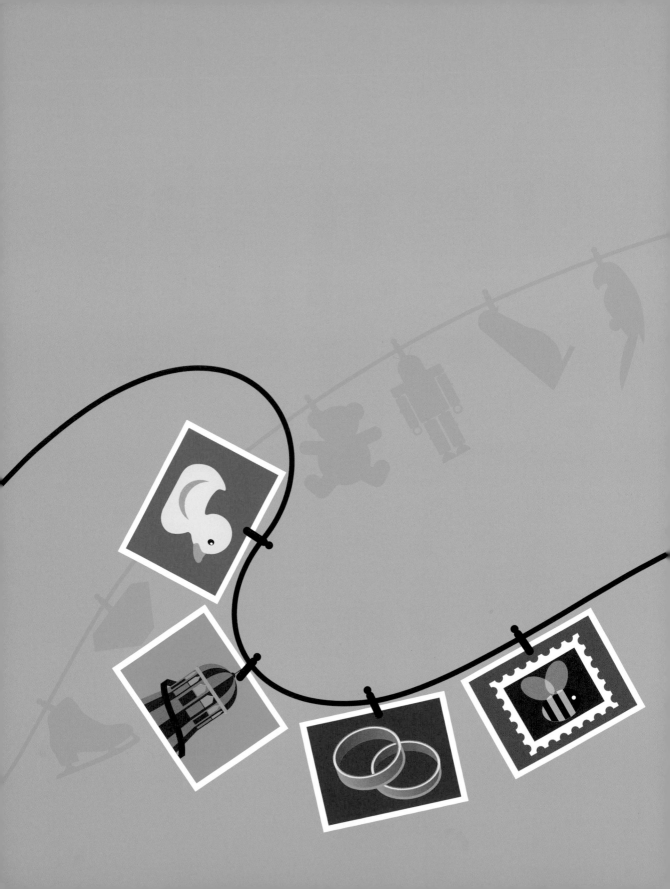

CHAPTER 3
IMPRINTING IT ON YOUR MIND
(LONG-TERM MEMORY)

Check-in: how well do you remember the past?

This chapter explores how long-term memory works and what you can do to improve it. Some exercises will ask you to retrieve memories from your own past while others will involve memorizing material and recalling it after a time-lag task.

1: Your life

Look back at your past and answer the following questions as accurately as possible. Leave the space blank if you cannot remember the answer.

▶ **A:** Where were you on Sunday a week ago?

▶ **B:** What was the name of your secondary school?

▶ **C:** What color hair does your dentist have?

▶ **D:** What was your previous address?

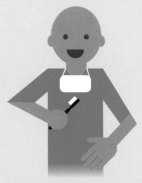

Your Score: _____
1 point for each correct answer

2: Dining with the famous

A genie has granted you a wish to have dinner with 8 world-famous people (past and present). Write down on their plates what each person is famous for.

Your Score: _____
1–4 correct: 2 points
5–8 correct: 4 points

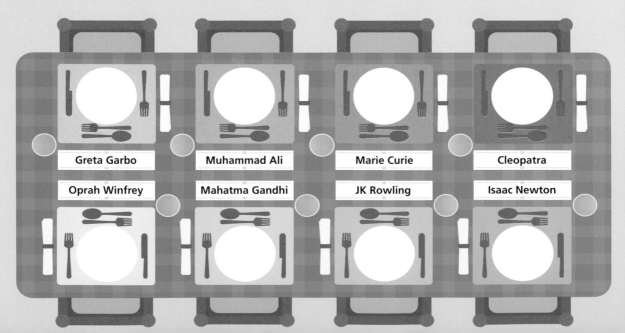

Greta Garbo

Muhammad Ali

Marie Curie

Cleopatra

Oprah Winfrey

Mahatma Gandhi

JK Rowling

Isaac Newton

3: Visual memories

How attentive are you? Try to answer the questions below using your visual memory of each object.

▶ **A:** How many wings do dragonflies have?

▶ **B:** Is the width of a credit card greater than 3 in?

▶ **C:** How many arrowheads does the universal recycling logo have?

▶ **D:** In Michelangelo's painting, *Creation of Adam*, which hand is Adam using to reach out to God?

▶ **E:** A standard ruler measures up to how many inches?

▶ **F:** Which colors make up the flag of the UK?

▶ **G:** What is the diameter of an adult human eye?

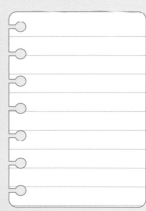

Solutions on p.181 ⟫

4: Weekly shopping

Here is your food-shopping list. Will you be able to bring back all these items? Study the list for a few minutes. Then cover it up and name 12 countries in Asia. (This will provide the time lag.) Afterward, try to recall as many items as possible. Write them down in the space provided.

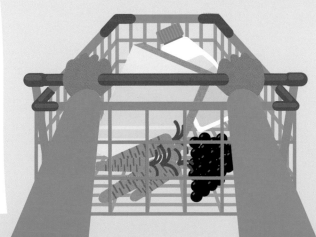

Carrots, Cookies,
Milk, Leeks, Pears,
Tape, Cheese,
Sausages,
Envelopes, Eggs,
Tomatoes, Wine,
Grapes, Cereals,
Ham

5: Closet crisis

You are trying to help your friend reorganize her closet after a dress-up session. Below (left) is what the closet originally looked like. Study it carefully for a few minutes and then cover it up. Now take a minute to recite the 13 times table. Afterward, return to the exercise—making sure the closet on the left is still covered up—and draw arrows to show where the items were originally located.

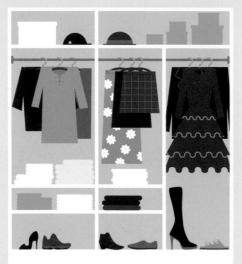

Your Score: _____
1–3 objects: 2 points
4–6 objects: 3 points
7–8 objects: 4 points
9–10 objects: 6 points

6: What were the questions?

The first exercise in this section asked you 4 questions about your life. Do you remember any of these questions? Write down as many as you can recall.

Your Score: _____
1 question: 1 point
2 questions: 2 points
3–4 questions: 4 points

7: Dog-sitting

You've offered to look after your friend's 3 dogs while she's away on vacation. When your friend brings the dogs to your house, she describes each one's personality for you. Take a few minutes to memorize the character traits of each dog and then cover up the words. Now to create time lag, spell out loud the first names of 8 family members. Afterward, try to write the traits of the 3 dogs in the answer spaces below.

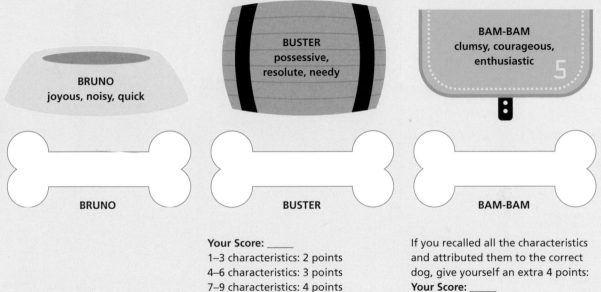

BRUNO
joyous, noisy, quick

BUSTER
possessive, resolute, needy

BAM-BAM
clumsy, courageous, enthusiastic

BRUNO   BUSTER   BAM-BAM

Your Score: _____
1–3 characteristics: 2 points
4–6 characteristics: 3 points
7–9 characteristics: 4 points

If you recalled all the characteristics and attributed them to the correct dog, give yourself an extra 4 points:
Your Score: _____

8: Shoes galore

Study these 16 types of footwear for a few minutes. Then cover up the picture and name 10 of your favorite cartoon characters to create a time lag. Afterward, write down as many styles as you can recall.

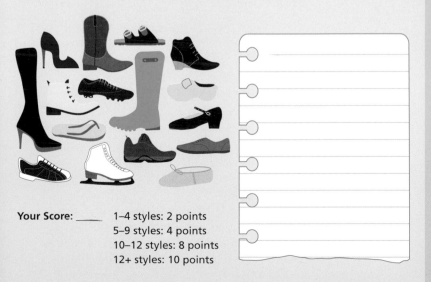

Your Score: _____   1–4 styles: 2 points
5–9 styles: 4 points
10–12 styles: 8 points
12+ styles: 10 points

HOW DID YOU DO?
Time to add up your points.
Your score: _____ ÷ **48 points**
= (_____ **x 100**) = _____ **%**
Did you fare better than you thought you would? You probably noticed that to complete these exercises, you could not rely on your short-term memory. In other words, you could not keep the information in your mental workspace because it was interrupted by another set of information during the time lag. So you had to sift through your long-term memory. Turn over to discover how your long-term memory works and discover ways to boost its aptitude.

What is long-term memory?

The image you have of your favorite schoolteacher, what you ate for breakfast this morning, and what you were doing 10 minutes ago are all in your long-term memory. Any memorized event that occurred outside the time limit of your short-term memory, which ranges from a few seconds to a minute, is in your long-term memory.

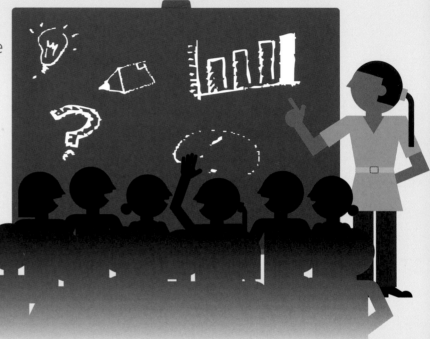

The two types

How many legs do flies have? What is the name of the secondary school you went to? You can probably recall that flies, like all insects, have six legs. You can probably name your old school quite easily, too. Although both these pieces of information are stored in your long-term memory, their nature is different: one is general knowledge, and you probably do not remember the context in which you learned it; the other is autobiographical and there are probably lots of emotions and other contextual memories attached to it.

The first type of information is called "semantic," and the second type is known as "episodic." A semantic memory is recalled as an isolated fact. In contrast, when an episodic memory is recalled, the person usually travels back in time and reexperiences the specific life episode along with the sensations attached to it.

The role of the hippocampus

All memories start as episodic memories. Over time, the context in which some were formed fades away and the memories become semantic.

The hippocampus (see p.14), which is a structure deep inside the temporal lobes of the brain, plays a crucial part in the formation of new episodic memories. Interestingly, some researchers believe that episodic memories are stored in the hippocampus, while others believe that it only stores episodic memories for a short time, after which the memories are consolidated to another part of the brain.

Are you ready to put your long-term memory to the test and try to recall some semantic and episodic memories? How about trying the two exercises on the opposite page?

9: Trip down memory lane

Write down 3 special moments from your childhood, 3 from your teenage years, and 3 from your adult life. Do you remember these moments like episodes of a favorite TV program, with the different people involved, the locations in which they took place, and the emotions you were feeling at the time?

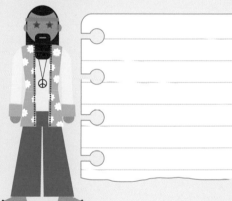

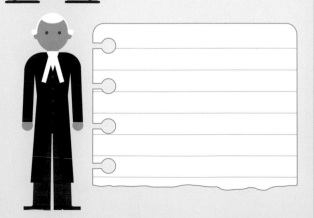

10: Where did I learn that?

Can you remember where you were and the source from which you learned the following pieces of information (e.g. a friend, television, newspaper, internet):

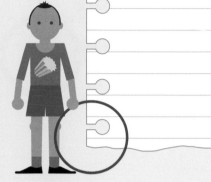

▶ **A:** The Statue of Liberty is in New York

▶ **B:** Mixing blue and yellow creates the color green

▶ **C:** Blueberries are a good source of antioxidants

▶ **D:** Elephants are known to have good memories

All the questions above tested your semantic memory, so the chances are you had trouble trying to figure out where and from whom you learned each piece of information.

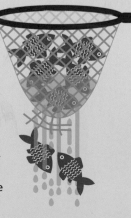

HOW IT WORKS: AMNESIA Long-term and short-term memories are independent and rely on different brain structures. For instance, people with total amnesia cannot register and/or retrieve long-term memories. They cannot learn new things, and cannot remember what happened five years or even five minutes ago. However, in some cases, the short-term memory is intact, enabling the person to hold information in their mind for a few seconds and manage tasks such as simple mental arithmetic.

Why do you never forget how to ride a bike?

Procedural, or "skill," memory is another type of long-term memory. This is the memory you use, for example, when you're riding a bike, playing a musical instrument, or doing a video game. It is the memory for how to do practical things. We are all born with an instinctive ability to form procedural memories. It is how we learn to eat, walk, and talk.

Practice is key

Any procedural memory is developed through practice, and depends on different brain structures from the ones supporting memories, which can be communicated verbally. Once you develop a practical skill, you can apply it automatically. This means that when called upon, you retrieve it without the need for conscious attention. The memory for practical skills is also very long-lasting. How about trying the following exercises to develop two different practical skills?

11: Play that tune

The sequence of musical notes on the right corresponds to the tune for the opening line of "Happy birthday." Practice on the portion of the piano below until you get the sequence right. Make sure you use the correct fingers, too. Try it out next time you come across a real piano!

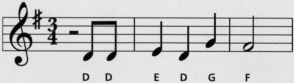

D D   E D G F

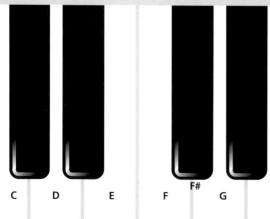

C   D   E   F   F#   G

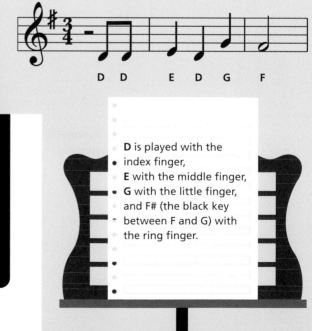

D is played with the index finger, E with the middle finger, G with the little finger, and F# (the black key between F and G) with the ring finger.

12: 3- and 4-strand braids

▶ **A:** Have you ever braided your own or somebody else's hair? This is a good example of a skill that stays with you forever once you have learned it.

Here is how you make a 3-strand braid. Practice with hair or threads until you can do it without thinking.

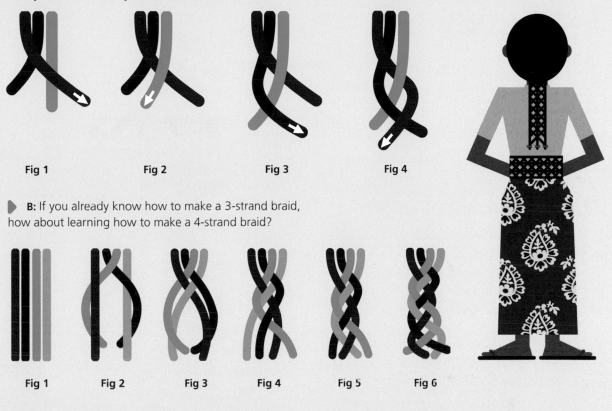

Fig 1   Fig 2   Fig 3   Fig 4

▶ **B:** If you already know how to make a 3-strand braid, how about learning how to make a 4-strand braid?

Fig 1   Fig 2   Fig 3   Fig 4   Fig 5   Fig 6

TOP TIP: HOW TO AVOID CHOKING UNDER PRESSURE Skills in procedural memory are practiced so often that they become automatic. However, pressure can cause even a skilled performer to falter. You sometimes see this happen in a professional sport when a player starts making simple mistakes and ends up losing from a seemingly unassailable position. Choking under pressure is caused by concentrating too hard on trying to monitor an automatic skill. This is counterproductive because the brain structures underlying skill memory are not consciously accessible. A way to avoid choking is to practice under simulated pressure situations: the brain will then gradually adapt to the conditions and stop focusing on the skill. This will then alleviate excessive stress and allow your procedural memory to function naturally.

SUPER TECHNIQUE:

How to boost memory of past events

"Curiosity is as much the parent of attention, as attention is of memory." These were the wise words of Richard Whately—educator, logician, and archbishop of Dublin in the 19th century— and form the basis of this technique.

The right frame of mind

If you didn't pay much attention to the details of the newspaper article you read this morning, the phone number of your doctor, or the name of the woman you met in yesterday's meeting, you probably won't be able to recollect any of these pieces of information. Is this such a surprise? You probably skimmed the article because it wasn't very interesting, you have your doctor's phone number on autodial so never need to look at the number, and you'll probably never meet that woman again.

   In short, we remember what we pay attention to, what we find interesting and surprising, what is important to us, and what has an emotional value (positive or negative). For example, a hobby that we are passionate about captures all of these things.

Memorability factor

Unfortunately, there are things we need to remember that do not possess these "hooks," such as the name of a medicine we have to take as well as the number of teaspoons, or the last place where we left our keys or reading glasses. The trick is to try to make day-to-day things such as these more memorable. This becomes possible when you apply the three key principles listed on the next page.

DID YOU KNOW: THE ACUTE MEMORIES OF SWAZI HERDSMEN

Can you recall what you bought for your dinner on the same day last month? Probably not. How about this then: herdsmen of the Swazi tribe of East Africa are able to remember in great detail each cow/bull purchased a year ago, including who sold the animal, whether it was a bull, a cow, or a calf, its age and look, and what it was bartered for. Impressive, huh? Cattle have tremendous social and economic importance in the Swazi tribe. When the psychologist Barlett tested the same men on other kinds of detail, their memory wasn't better than the average person's. The conclusion we can draw from this is that we generally remember stuff that matters most to us!

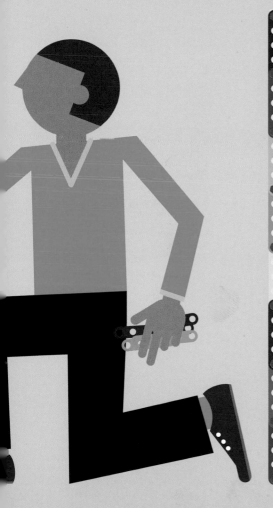

The key principles

Be attentive Although this seems obvious, paying attention to what you want to memorize is the first step toward successfully recalling it. For example, when you cannot remember where you last put your keys, your memory is not at fault. Most of the time this happens because you did not pay attention to where you placed them in the first place. The brain cannot retrieve information that it has not registered.

Be curious Memories that are rich in emotion and connected with many others are much easier to recall. Curiosity will help you create richer memories. By being curious, you will create connections between new and past events: you will feel more involved and this will trigger emotions. For instance, asking people questions about what they do and things they like will help you remember them and their names. Wondering how a medicine works may help you remember its name.

Be motivated Putting a concerted effort into memorizing plays a key role in how well you are able to retrieve a piece of information. Improving memory is like improving any skill. To master it requires continuous practice. It is not easy, but it can be done!

Create personal meaning

A married couple never forgets the memory of their wedding day, especially the moment they exchange the marriage vows and then, of course, the rings. This is because the occasion is full of personal meaning, which naturally commands attention, curiosity, and motivation—the key principles we've already discussed. To improve your memory for random pieces of information, you can attach personal meaning to them. Try exercise 13 below to see how applying this method can help with memorization.

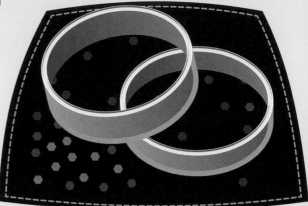

13: It's mine!

Below are pictures of 12 objects that most people use on a regular basis. How many of these objects do you think you will be able to memorize in just over a minute?

For each object, think about the one you have at home and where it is located. Spend 5 seconds developing a personal association with each object. When you are done, cover up the pictures. Then, to create a time lag, complete the math problems on the right. Afterward, return to the exercise and list as many objects as you can recall.

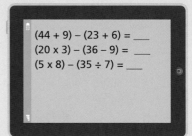

(44 + 9) – (23 + 6) = ___
(20 x 3) – (36 – 9) = ___
(5 x 8) – (35 ÷ 7) = ___

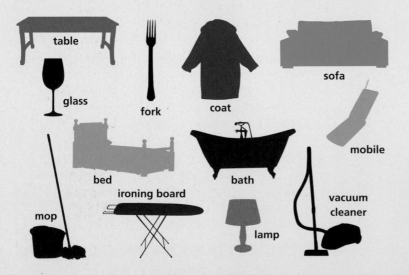

table

glass

fork

coat

sofa

mobile

bed

ironing board

bath

mop

lamp

vacuum cleaner

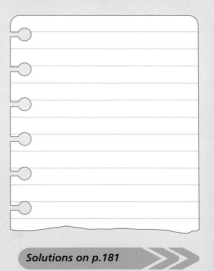

Solutions on p.181 ▶▶▶

14: Memorable day

Most of us are creatures of habit and our lives are bound by routine. This explains why what we did last Monday can be difficult to recall. To counter this, how about organizing a memorable day? You could take part in a unique activity that is enjoyable and meaningful to you.

Here are some ideas: go for a walk in an unfamiliar setting, buy something unusual for yourself or someone else, have coffee with a friend at a new venue, take a class in something novel, or visit a fun-packed place such as a carnival with friends or family.

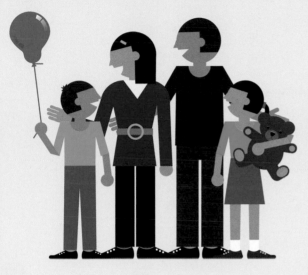

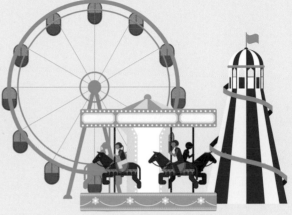

15: Your favorite song

Listen to a song that used to be a favorite when you were a teenager. You might be surprised by how evocative this is and how long-forgotten emotions associated with the memories come flooding back. Write down the details and feelings that return to you.

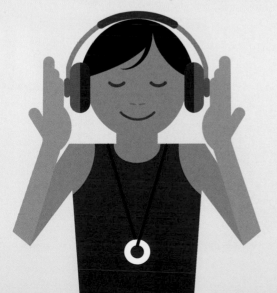

DID YOU KNOW: FLASHBULB MEMORIES Do you remember how you spent New Year's Eve in 1999? Cast your mind back to the eve of the millennium, the place, and the people you were with. Your memory of this is probably quite vivid and rich in details. This is what is called a flashbulb memory: a precise, concrete, and long-lasting memory of the context surrounding a special event. (The event can be a shocking one, too, such as the moment you find out that something tragic has happened.) There are two reasons why such memories stick in your mind. Not only was the moment they were registered very emotional, but they also tend to be retold or relived over and over again.

Does learning by rote work?

At school most of us memorized by rote material such as poems and math formulas. Some of us still use this method to memorize information. Learning by rote is based on repetition. The idea is that the more you repeat something, the better the chance that it will stick in your mind.

Limitations of rote-learning

Going over a piece of information several times does increase the likelihood of remembering it. The major problem with this technique is that it doesn't require you to understand what you are learning. If the memorized information is not well understood, it will not become connected to existing knowledge (concepts) and, therefore, will be harder to retrieve later on. This explains why material memorized by rote is often forgotten if it is not rehearsed frequently. The perfect example is a student who crams information just before an exam, but doesn't remember much of it a few months later.

Self-testing

Meaningful learning, in which the new information is understood and connected to existing knowledge, usually leads to better and longer-lasting memories. Another effective learning method is known as "self-testing." When using this method, you test your memory several times at regular intervals for the facts you want to memorize, either on the same day or on different days. After you've tried to recall the information, you check the accuracy of your recall by looking at the original facts. Self-testing is more effective than rote-learning, and a better way of training your brain to recall. Try the following exercise.

16: Rote-learning vs self-testing

You want to remember the facts below for a game show in which you will appear as a contestant in a week's time. Use rote-learning to learn the first 3 facts: repeat each fact out loud 10 times. Afterward, use the self-testing method to learn the remaining 3 facts over the period of a day. Re-read the facts, and then test yourself again later in the day. Continue to do this until you can recall the 3 facts without making a single error. Try to recall all 6 facts in 2 days' time (making sure the facts are covered up).

- As of 2009, there were 528 million people living on the North American continent.
- In the UK, the life expectancy of men is 77.6 years, and and of women, 81.7 years.
- The atmosphere on Venus is composed primarily of carbon dioxide.
- An oxymoron is the juxtaposition of two contradictory words (for example, a deafening silence).
- As of 2005, 34 percent of the population age 15 and over in Algeria was illiterate.
- The world track record for the 1-mile competition is held by a Moroccan athlete who ran it in 3 minutes 43 seconds in 1999.

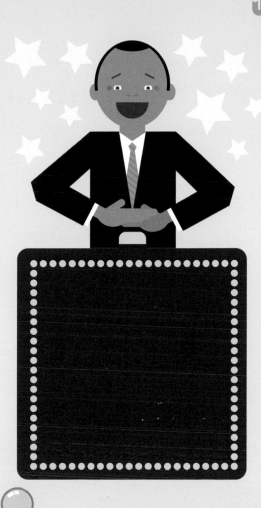

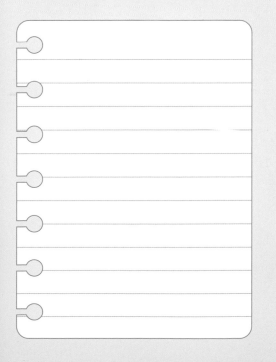

DID YOU KNOW: ROTE-LEARNING OR PARROT FASHION? Different countries use a variety of colorful terms to refer to rote-learning. In Greece, rote-learning is known as *papagalia* "parrot-like learning," while in France it is called *par cœur* "by heart." It is not highly regarded in either country, where teachers tend to prefer comprehension instead. In parts of China, it is known as *tian yazi* "stuff the duck," while in Germany it is called *Der Nürnberger Trichter* "the Nuremberg Funnel," in both cases suggesting that knowledge is simply pushed into the student. However, China does consider rote-learning to be an integral part of its teaching culture.

Check-out: exercise your long-term memory

Now that you're familiar with the principles for effective memorizing, it's time to assess your long-term memory skills. Calculate your score for each exercise. Remember to be attentive and curious throughout. Some of the exercises will ask you to memorize information and then recall it after a delay or a time-lag task.

17: Panic at the toy store!

All the toys have been mixed up! Can you put them back where they belong? Study the diagram below showing which toys belong in which bucket. Then cover up the diagram. Before sorting the toys, take a minute to solve the math problems below. Afterward, sort the toys by writing the letter of the correct bin next to each one.

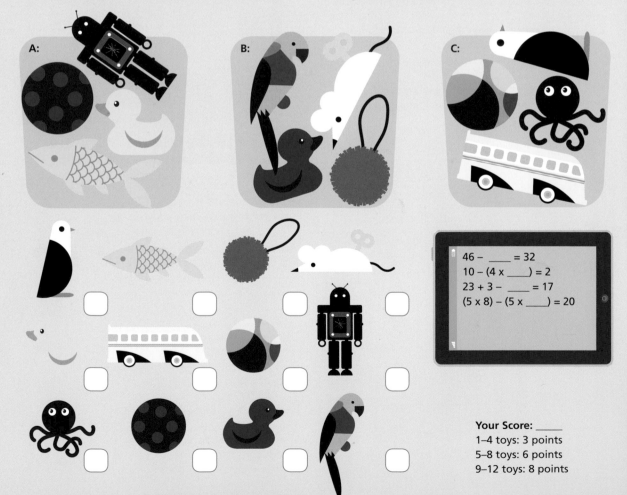

$$46 - \rule{1cm}{0.15mm} = 32$$
$$10 - (4 \times \rule{1cm}{0.15mm}) = 2$$
$$23 + 3 - \rule{1cm}{0.15mm} = 17$$
$$(5 \times 8) - (5 \times \rule{1cm}{0.15mm}) = 20$$

Your Score: _____
1–4 toys: 3 points
5–8 toys: 6 points
9–12 toys: 8 points

18: Martian invasion

You're trying to read this old newspaper clipping. Some of the words have faded and are illegible. Can you figure out what the words that are missing should be? Cover the text when you are done. Then take a minute to recall the facts you learned in exercise 16 on page 67. Now write down as many of the missing words as you can recall, making sure the words you filled in in the first place are still covered up.

You may find that the easier it was to fill in the blank, the less attention you paid to the word and, probably, the more difficult it was to recall it.

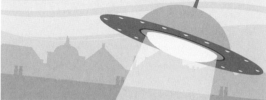

Latest _____: a large Martian _____ is confirmed. The first spacecrafts were _____ this _____ over Spain and France. Further reports indicate that the fleet is heading toward Great _____. In London, the streets are filling up with _____ citizens gazing at the sky. _____ are full as people are trying to buy anything they can before the invasion. Cars and _____ are lining up on the main _____. Traveling may become _____ in a few hours.

Solutions on p.181

Your Score: _____   1–3 words: 3 points
4–7 words: 6 points
8–10 words: 8 points

19: Origami puppy face

Have you ever tried origami, the Japanese craft of paper folding? Let's give it a try. Take 5 minutes to memorize the step-by-step instructions to create an origami puppy face. Use the illustrations to visualize each fold. Then close the book and get a square piece of paper. Now can you fold from memory?

Your Score: _____
1–2 folds: 3 points
3–4 folds: 4 points
5 folds: 6 points

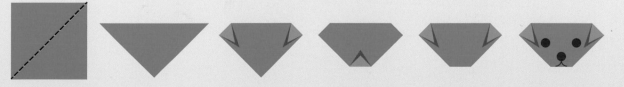

1. Fold along the diagonal to get a triangle, then fold the triangle in half to make a smaller triangle.

2. Hold the triangle with the point facing down and fold the 2 corners down. These are your dog's ears.

3. Turn the paper over and fold the tip of the triangle inward.

4. Turn the paper over and draw 2 eyes, a nose, and a mouth.

20: Facing the enemies

Below are the different types of aliens that you will encounter in a video game. Your first job is to make sure you know which ones are your friends and which ones are the enemies. Study them carefully for several minutes. When you are done, cover up the chart. Then take a minute to solve the word puzzle on the right. Afterward, on the second chart, mark a check beside the friendly aliens and an "x" by the enemies.

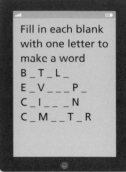

Fill in each blank with one letter to make a word
B _ T _ L _
E _ V _ _ _ P _
C _ I _ _ _ N
C _ M _ _ T _ R

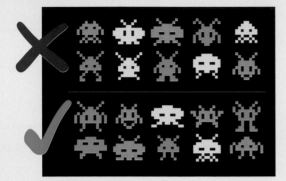

Your Score: _____
1–5 aliens: 4 points
6–10 aliens: 8 points
10–15 aliens: 12 points
16–20 aliens: 15 points

21: Eyewitness

Have you ever wondered how accurate you would be if you were asked questions about a scene you had just witnessed? Let's give it a try. Study this scene for a few minutes. Then cover it up and take a few minutes to solve the math problems. Afterward, answer the questions below.

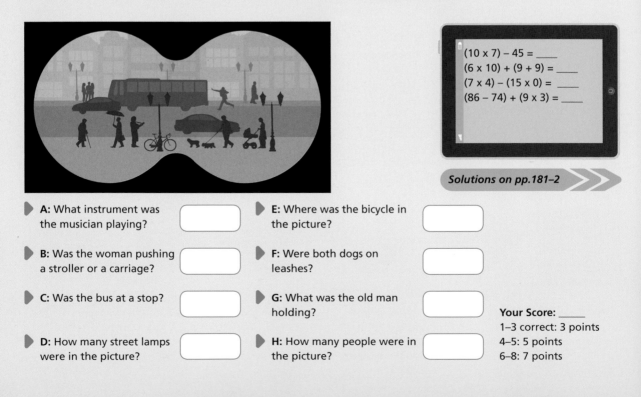

$(10 \times 7) - 45 =$ _____
$(6 \times 10) + (9 + 9) =$ _____
$(7 \times 4) - (15 \times 0) =$ _____
$(86 - 74) + (9 \times 3) =$ _____

Solutions on pp.181–2 ⟩⟩⟩

▶ **A:** What instrument was the musician playing?

▶ **B:** Was the woman pushing a stroller or a carriage?

▶ **C:** Was the bus at a stop?

▶ **D:** How many street lamps were in the picture?

▶ **E:** Where was the bicycle in the picture?

▶ **F:** Were both dogs on leashes?

▶ **G:** What was the old man holding?

▶ **H:** How many people were in the picture?

Your Score: _____
1–3 correct: 3 points
4–5: 5 points
6–8: 7 points

22: Reading a map

You are getting ready for a long trip across Europe. Below is your itinerary. Study it for a few minutes and then cover it up. Take a 2-minute break Afterward, trace your route on the map below.

Your Score: _____
1–3 cities: 3 points
4–6 cities: 6 points
7–8 cities: 8 points

Your itinerary:
Start in Paris (France),
then to Bern (Switzerland),
Florence (Italy), Rome
(Italy), Vienna (Austria),
Munich (Germany), Bonn
(Germany), Rotterdam
(Netherlands), and
back to Paris

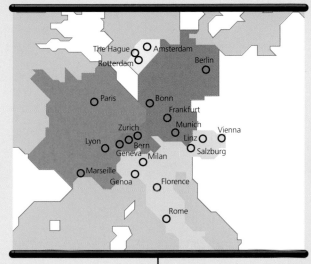

23: The "visiting girls" ceremony

Read the passage below, cover it up, then take a minute's break before answering the questions below.

The Dai people of China practice an annual courtship ritual called "visiting girls." It starts out with young women sitting around a bonfire and turning their spinning wheels. They are approached by a group of men draped in red blankets who are playing musical instruments. Each man chooses a woman to serenade. If the woman of his choice finds him attractive, she'll take out a small stool from under her skirt and invite him to sit on it. Then the man will wrap her in his red blanket.

A: In which country does the ceremony take place?

B: How often does the ceremony occur?

C: What do the young men do?

D: What do the men wear?

E: What do the women keep under their skirts?

F: How do the women express their interest to the men?

Your Score: _____
1–2 questions: 1 point
3–4 questions: 3 points
5–6 questions: 8 points

24: Moments from the past

Answer these questions accurately. Put an "x" in the box if you don't know the answer:

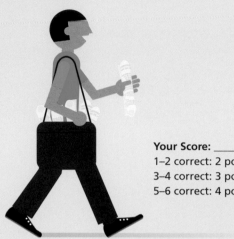

A: What was your telephone number at your last address?

B: What was your first job?

C: What did you do on Saturday night two weeks ago?

D: Can you name one of your primary school teachers.

E: What was the title of the last book you read?

F: What is the eye color of your dentist?

Your Score: _____
1–2 correct: 2 points
3–4 correct: 3 points
5–6 correct: 4 points

25: First glimpse of the ocean

Your friend is describing the first time he saw the ocean while on vacation. Try to visualize the scene as you read the postcard. When you are done, cover it up and recall the names of 10 people who were in your class in secondary school. Afterward, draw what you remember of the scene.

Your Score: _____
1–3 correctly located objects: 3 points
4–6 objects: 5 points
7–10+ objects: 8 points

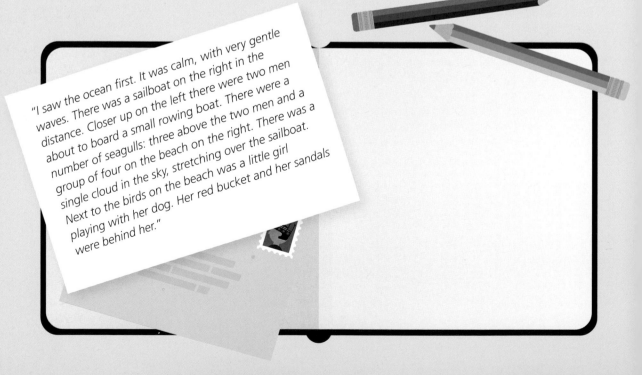

"I saw the ocean first. It was calm, with very gentle waves. There was a sailboat on the right in the distance. Closer up on the left there were two men about to board a small rowing boat. There were a number of seagulls: three above the two men and a group of four on the beach on the right. There was a single cloud in the sky, stretching over the sailboat. Next to the birds on the beach was a little girl playing with her dog. Her red bucket and her sandals were behind her."

26: Birthday wish

You accidentally spill water on your god-daughter's birthday wish list. The words become illegible so you try to remember what they were. Study this wish list for a few minutes. To create richer memories, try to think of each item in a personal context. Then cover up the list and try to find your way in the maze on the right. Afterward, rewrite the list on the blank sheet below and see how many items you can remember.

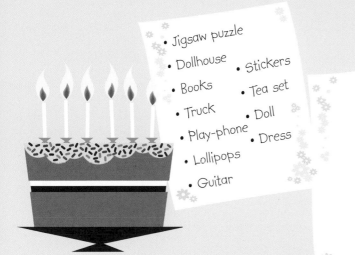

- Jigsaw puzzle
- Dollhouse
- Stickers
- Books
- Tea set
- Truck
- Doll
- Play-phone
- Dress
- Lollipops
- Guitar

Your Score: _____
1–4 items: 3 points
5–8 items: 6 points
9–11 items: 8 points

27: Follow the recipe

You're tired of referring back to your cookbook to remember the ingredients you need for a recipe. How about trying to memorize them instead? Take 2 minutes to study the list of ingredients, then cover it up, and complete the time-lag task on the right. Now draw a circle around the ingredients you need.

The formula to convert °C to °F is:
°F = (°C x ⅗) + 32°
How many degrees Fahrenheit does 218°F convert to? _____

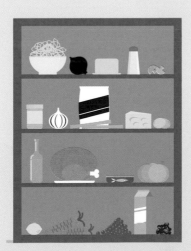

butter, onion,
pasta, celery,
mushrooms,
flour, salt,
milk, tuna,
peas, cheese

Solutions on p.182

Your Score: _____
1–4 ingredients: 3 points
5–8 ingredients: 6 points
9–11 ingredients: 8 points

28: Geography lesson

How much do you remember from your geography lessons at school?
Draw arrows to link each river with the sea or ocean it flows into.

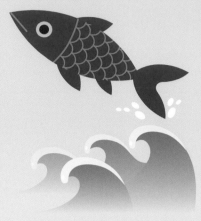

River
A: Mississippi
B: Jordan
C: Seine
D: Ganges
E: Danube
F: Euphrates
G: Amazon
H: Mekong

Ocean/Sea
South China Sea
English Channel
Dead Sea
Atlantic Ocean
Persian Gulf
Black Sea
Indian Ocean
Gulf of Mexico

Your Score: _____
1 point for each correct
answer

Solutions on p.182

29: Who said what?

You are having dinner with new colleagues and they all tell you something about
themselves. Take a few minutes to memorize each statement and the face it belongs
to. Then cover up the picture. After a 5-minute break, write the correct statement in
each speech bubble.

Your Score: _____
1–2 quotes: 3 points
3–4 quotes: 6 points
5–6 quotes: 8 points

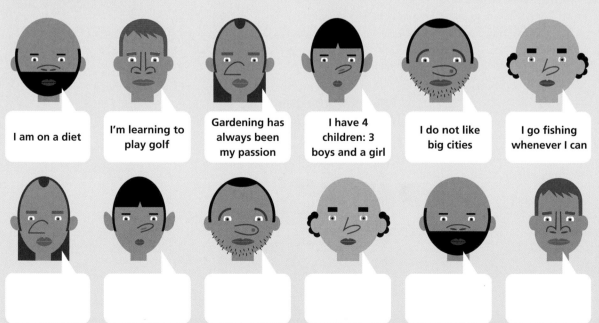

30: All mixed up!

At a conference, you bump into a colleague and all the business cards you both have collected fall on the floor and get mixed up. Take a few minutes to memorize the names on the business cards in the holder. Then cover them up. Now, to create a time lag, recall the 8 Wonders of the World. Afterward, identify your business cards from the pile.

Your Score: _____
1–2 cards: 3 points
3–4 cards: 6 points
5–6 cards: 8 points

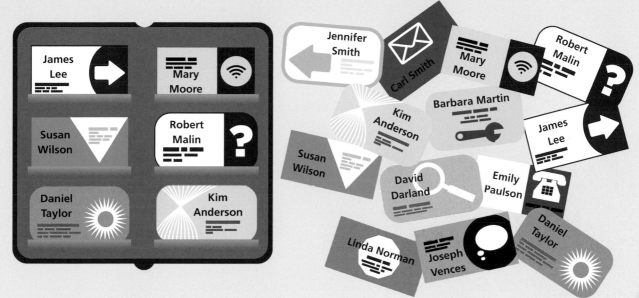

31: Stamp collector

You've spotted 10 stamps that you think may interest your friend who is an avid stamp collector. However, you're not sure whether he already has them. Take a few minutes to memorize the 10 stamps below (on the left). Then, to create a time lag, turn back to pages 72–73 and add up your score for the exercises on those 2 pages. Afterward, return to this exercise (making sure the stamps you studied are covered up). Study your friend's collection and cross off the stamps that you have spotted that your friend already has.

1 0

HOW DID YOU DO?
Time to add up your points.
Your score: _____ ÷ **122 points**
= (_____ x 100) = _____ %
Compare this score to the score you got for the check-in exercises. Are they different? How much were you able to focus your attention and create rich memories?

Do bear in mind that you cannot improve your memory over the course of a single day! What you can do is maintain the good work and make sure you keep applying the basic principles described in this chapter as often as possible when trying to memorize something.

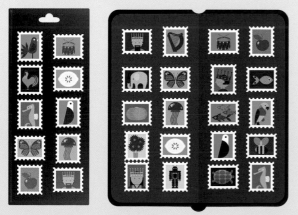

Your Score: _____
1–2 stamps: 3 points
3–4 stamps: 6 points
5–6 stamps: 8 points
7 stamps: 10 points

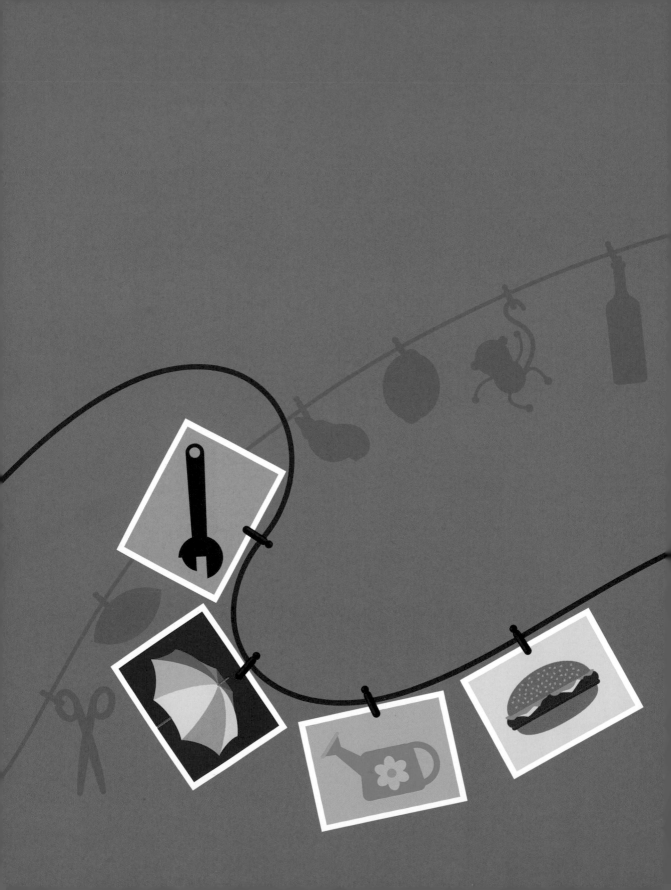

CHAPTER 4

LEAVING A VIVID IMPRESSION ON YOUR MIND
(MEMORY AND IMAGINATION)

Check-in: what's your imagination like?

Recall a special moment in your life. Do images of the moment come to mind first? Of course they do. This is because we rely mainly on our sense of vision to build memories in the first place. This chapter looks at how honing the ability to create powerful mental images can lead to a better memory. Try the following exercises to assess your visualization skills.

1: Close your eyes to see

Visualize the following images and then rate the vividness of each image on a scale of 1 to 4:

1 = vague impression
2 = complete but lacking detail
3 = complete with a few details
4 = vivid impression

▶ **A:** Your mother's face. Your rating: ____

▶ **B:** A market stall. Your rating: ____

▶ **C:** The sun setting behind a mountain. Your rating: ____

▶ **D:** A cat warming up in the sun. Your rating: ____

▶ **E:** A forest in fall. Your rating: ____

▶ **F:** A sailboat on a rough sea. Your rating: ____

What is your average rating (sum of all your ratings divided by 6)? Your Score: _____

2: What happens next?

Look at each scene and try to imagine what will happen next. You can either draw or describe the next scene in the space provided. Try to imagine something funny or surprising. You have 2 minutes.

Your score: _____
1 scene: 3 points
2 scenes: 6 points

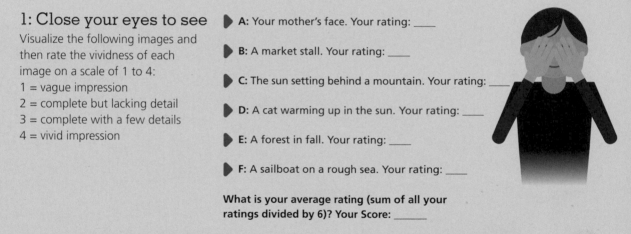

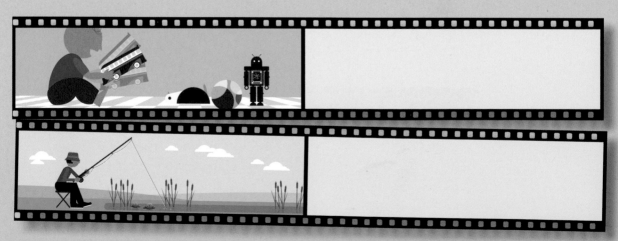

3: Back to front

Choose a room in your house (not the one you're currently in), and imagine all the furniture mirrored so that what's on the left is now on the right and vice versa. Draw an aerial plan of the mirrored room in the space below. Then go to that room and check how accurate your drawing is.

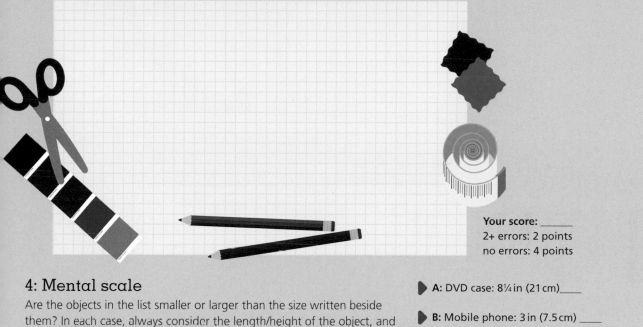

Your score: _____
2+ errors: 2 points
no errors: 4 points

4: Mental scale

Are the objects in the list smaller or larger than the size written beside them? In each case, always consider the length/height of the object, and NOT the width. Write "S" (smaller) or "L" (larger) beside each object.

▶ **A:** DVD case: 8¼ in (21 cm)_____

▶ **B:** Mobile phone: 3 in (7.5 cm) _____

▶ **C:** Checkbook: 2⅓ in (6 cm) _____

▶ **D:** Ballpoint pen: 3½ in (9 cm)_____

▶ **E:** Wine bottle: 14¼ in (36 cm) _____

▶ **F:** Cotton swab: 2¾ in (7 cm)_____

▶ **G:** Fork: 9 in (23 cm)_____

▶ **H:** Coffee mug: 5⅓ in (13.5 cm)_____

▶ **I:** Business card: 1½ in (4 cm)_____

Your score: _____
1–3 correct: 2 points
4–6 correct: 4 points
7–9 correct: 6 points

Solutions on p.182

5: Tactile memories

Can you recall what it feels like to walk on a warm sandy beach? If the answer is yes, you've just experienced a "kinesthetic" image. In other words, you've just recalled the feeling you get when a part of your body touches something familiar.

How strong are your kinesthetic images? Imagine the following actions and rate how difficult it is to recall the feeling on a scale of 1–4:

1 = very difficult, 2 = difficult, 3 = moderately easy, 4 = easy

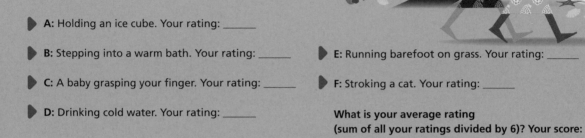

► **A:** Holding an ice cube. Your rating: _____

► **B:** Stepping into a warm bath. Your rating: _____

► **C:** A baby grasping your finger. Your rating: _____

► **D:** Drinking cold water. Your rating: _____

► **E:** Running barefoot on grass. Your rating: _____

► **F:** Stroking a cat. Your rating: _____

What is your average rating (sum of all your ratings divided by 6)? Your score: _____

6: Imaginary turns

How good are you at mentally rotating objects? Let's give it a try. By mentally turning them left or right, decide whether the objects in each pair below are identical (I) or mirrored (M) images.

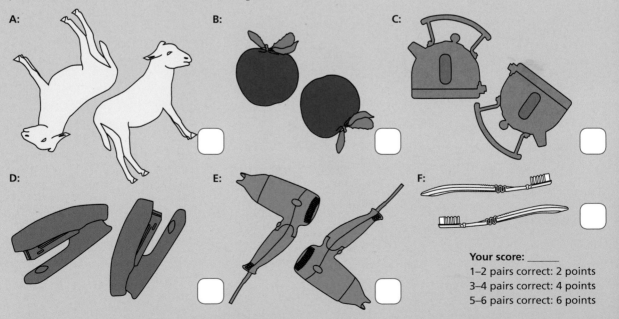

A:

B:

C:

D:

E:

F:

Your score: _____
1–2 pairs correct: 2 points
3–4 pairs correct: 4 points
5–6 pairs correct: 6 points

7: It's all in the detail

How precise are your mental images? Search your memory to answer the following questions.

▶ **A:** Do bears have short or long tails?

▶ **B:** What color is the inside of a mango?

▶ **C:** Are flamingos pink all over?

▶ **D:** What's the color of an uncooked shrimp?

▶ **E:** Do bats have large or small ears?

▶ **F:** What does the shape of Italy remind you of?

Your score: _____
1 point for each correct answer

Solutions on p.182 ▷▷▷

8: Zooming in

A butterfly appears bigger as you get closer to it, right? This can be experienced mentally, too. Imagine a butterfly on a flower 3 feet away from you and then begin zooming in on it. You can see the pattern on the wings. You may even be able to see its antennae and eyes. See, it works! Now imagine a caterpillar on a leaf 3 feet away from you. Zoom in on it and on a separate piece of paper list as many details as you can "see."

Your score: _____
1–3 details spotted: 2 points
4–6 details spotted: 3 points
7+ details spotted: 4 points

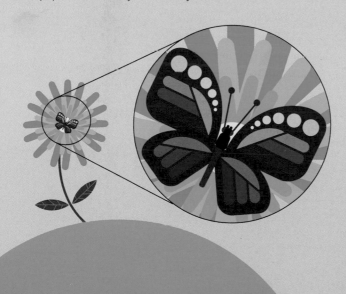

1 0

HOW DID YOU DO?
Time to add up your points.
Your score = (____ x 100) ÷ 40 = ____ %
Were you able to visualize images that were vividly detailed? Which aspect of visualization did you find the most challenging: color, size, or shape? During this chapter, you will find out why visualization is one of the keys to boosting memory. You will also learn 2 memory techniques that involve visualization.

How does visualization boost memory?

Pictures are more powerful than words to help retrieve a memory. This is because the brain registers pictures both at the conceptual and the visual level. For example, when you see a picture of a cheeseburger, you understand what it is (conceptual level) and you see what it looks like (visual level). In contrast, when you just hear the word "cheeseburger," you register it at the conceptual level and do not get any visual cues, so your brain has to work a little bit harder to access the memory.

The power of images

The superiority of images over words has been known for a long time. This is why most mnemonics boost your memory by asking you to convert what you want to learn into powerful mental images. The idea is that these images will stick in your mind because the brain registers them at both conceptual and visual levels, just as real pictures.

Mental images also help you create connections between the different things you want to remember. For instance, if you want to memorize that your new neighbor has a white cat as well as a toddler child, try to picture both in a single image—you can imagine the cat licking the toddler's hand or the toddler riding the cat! Such images might seem silly, but they are very powerful memory boosters.

Using the other senses

When you recall an object in your mind, you form a mental image of it, but you can also recall other sensory experiences of the object. For instance, if you're asked to think about chocolate, you probably begin by picturing your favorite chocolate bar, the packaging it's in, but then you can also imagine its smell, what it feels like on your fingers, and of course its taste when you put it into your mouth.

One way to create strong memories is to form images and enrich them with multisensory details. This will increase your chances of retrieving the memory. As with all the techniques featured in this book, the more you practice this multisensory technique, the better you will become at using it, and it will soon become a memory aid that you employ without even having to think about it.

9: Pictures and words

Take a few minutes to memorize the group of pictures and the list of words. When you are done, cover them up. Then, to make sure that none of these are present in your short-term memory, recite the 8 multiplication table backward starting from 80. Afterward, write down the pictures and words you can remember.

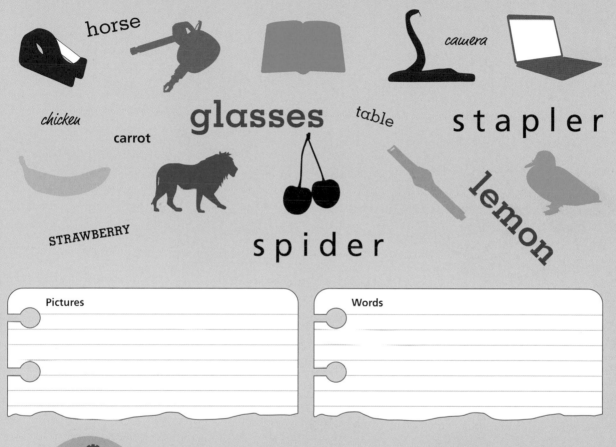

horse

camera

chicken

glasses

table

stapler

carrot

STRAWBERRY

spider

lemon

Pictures

Words

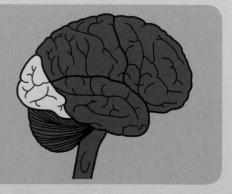

HOW IT WORKS: WHY ARE MY MENTAL IMAGES NOT VIVID?
Picture a child running after a multicolored ball. How is your mental image? Is it richly detailed, full of color, and as precise as a photograph? Or is it rather vague and dim? People report a lot of differences in the vividness of their mental images. Why is this? Research shows that the vividness of mental images is determined by the activity in the primary area of the brain which processes visual information (in the occipital lobe, at the back of your head). The more activity there is in this part of the brain, the more vivid your mental images.

How do special moments stick in your mind?

We tend to remember moments, events, or things that are different from what we usually encounter. Our first experience of something is a perfect example, such as the first day of school, the first time we drive a car, or the first time we share a romantic kiss. Why is this?

The power of emotion

Such salient events attract our attention. This extra attention leads to a better memory of the event because more information becomes registered in the brain, and this additional information acts as a cue for retrieval later on.

In addition, salient events can sometimes rouse emotional states of surprise, pleasure, or shock. For example, most of us have no problem recounting our first day of school because we felt extremely curious, excited, and apprehensive on that day. Our heightened emotions triggered a state of arousal in which we were more alert and attentive. As a result, more information was registered during this event. In contrast, it's perhaps far more difficult to recount the memory of our third day at school because, as we became accustomed to our new surroundings, our emotions settled down.

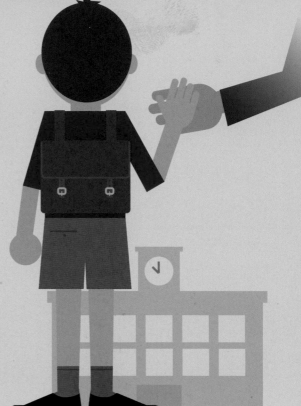

Adding humor

There are many memory-boosting techniques that take advantage of the power of uniqueness on memory. This is the case, for example, in the Link System (see pp.88–89), in which the person creates surprising and original mental images using the material they are trying to memorize. These mental images tend to be funny too. This is because humor stimulates our attention substantially. For instance, it is well known in the advertising world that humorous advertisements are more memorable than serious ones. In fact, the next time you're watching television, count the number of advertisements you see that use humor to sell their product. You'll be surprised how often the scene, narrative, or strapline relies on humor to attract your attention. So the funnier you can make your mental images when using visual mnemonics, the better your memory of them will be.

10: Funny images

Spend 1 minute studying the 6 pictures that are on the front page of the magazine below. Then cover up the image and complete the math problems in the time lag task. Afterward, write down as many objects as you can remember from the 6 drawings in the magazine.

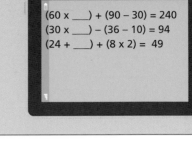

$(60 \times \underline{\quad}) + (90 - 30) = 240$
$(30 \times \underline{\quad}) - (36 - 10) = 94$
$(24 + \underline{\quad}) + (8 \times 2) = 49$

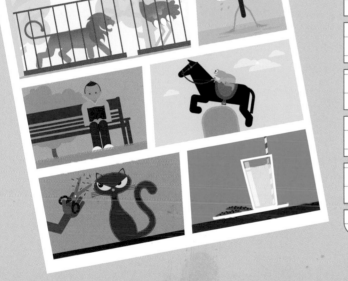

Did you recall the objects that featured in the funnier/bizarre images more easily than the objects in the ordinary images? It is likely that the funnier scenes made a greater impact and stuck in your mind. This demonstrates the power of humor and uniqueness in memory formation.

Solutions on p.182

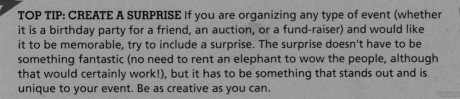

TOP TIP: CREATE A SURPRISE If you are organizing any type of event (whether it is a birthday party for a friend, an auction, or a fund-raiser) and would like it to be memorable, try to include a surprise. The surprise doesn't have to be something fantastic (no need to rent an elephant to wow the people, although that would certainly work!), but it has to be something that stands out and is unique to your event. Be as creative as you can.

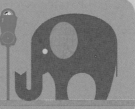

Why can't you get that song out of your head?

Do you remember the songs you used to sing as a child? And can you easily recall the words to the songs you listened to as a teenager? Can you remember the melody as well as the lyrics? It is likely that you answered yes to these questions. How is it that songs seem to stick easily in our memories? There are 3 main reasons for this: repetition, the emotion we invested in the songs while listening to them, and the meaning of particular songs.

Making songs stick

We tend to hear songs we like over and over again. The more we like them, the more we listen to them, and if we like them a lot we tend to sing along, especially in the shower! Knowingly or unknowingly, we rehearse our favorite songs extensively, which increases the likelihood that they will stay with us forever.

Another reason why songs sometimes find a permanent home in our memories is because they are registered at several levels in our brain. First, both music and lyrics can trigger emotion, be it pleasure, joy, optimism, or sadness. Secondly, the lyrics of a song may hold special meaning for us. They might tell a poignant story, or encapsulate perfectly the moment we first fell in love. The combination of melody and lyrics makes a song both emotive and expository. This makes the memory of a song a very rich one and therefore easier to retrieve later on.

Other benefits

The relationship between music and memory is complex. Not only do songs we like stick in our heads, but music can also help alleviate anxiety and stress. Since a high level of stress is not good for memory (see pp.168–169), music can be considered to be an indirect memory booster. Its relaxing effect helps us function better (although listening to music while studying may not be the smartest choice; see tip box opposite).

Interestingly, the context in which songs are heard often stays with us. This makes songs powerful tools to elicit autobiographical memories, especially when memory begins to decline with age.

Finally, because songs tend to stay in our memories for a while, they can be good tools to learn new facts. This can be achieved by replacing the lyrics of a well-known song with information you have to remember. Try the exercise "Singing to remember" on the next page to see how this works.

11: Singing to remember

You have 4 things to do today and decide to take advantage of the powerful effect of songs on memory to memorize your to-do list. You need a short and simple song. Let's pick a children's song that you probably know very well, such as "Frère Jacques."

Replace the lyrics of the song with the items on your to-do list. Sing the song several times with its new "lyrics." How fast can you learn the song (and thus memorize your list)? This also works very well when memorizing phone numbers, for example.

Frère Jacques (repeat)
Are you sleeping? (repeat)
Morning bells are ringing (repeat)
Ding Ding Dong (repeat)

Pay the water bill (repeat)
Buy some cheese (repeat)
Take shirt to dry cleaners (repeat)
Phone Aunt Sue (repeat)

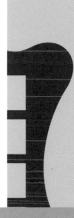

TOP TIP: NO MUSIC WHILE STUDYING! When you listen to music while reviewing for an exam, you're doing 2 things at the same time. This means that you are dividing your attention between the music and the material you are trying to learn. So you have less attention available for memorizing, which is likely to lead to poorer recall during the exam (see pp.62–63 to read more about attention and memory). It is therefore better to study in a quiet environment. If you miss the soothing effect of music too much, listen to music without lyrics, which is less likely to grab and divide your attention.

SUPER TECHNIQUE:

The Link System

A memory is rarely a single isolated fact. Most often it will be a collection of connected information. This is how learning happens in the brain: new facts are connected to old ones, and it is through this system of linkage that we store and retrieve information. This also explains why single facts, such as names, can be so difficult to remember.

We make natural connections

Sometimes connections form naturally when we encounter a new fact. For example, if your colleague tells you that he bought a new minivan, you will remember this because you can connect the information to something else you know about him, namely, that he has 4 kids so he needs a large car. Other times we come across isolated information and no connections come to mind. This might be the case when you meet Sally Kay for the first time. Your chances of remembering her name are slim without creating any connections. This is when the Link System (or association technique) comes in handy.

What is the Link System?

In the Link System, you use your imagination to create artificial links/connections/associations between random objects. The more creatively you use your imagination, the stronger the links will be. And the stronger the links, the better your memory of those objects will be. There are 2 key methods to create strong links:

Exaggeration: links that are larger than life, strange, funny, or surprising are always more memorable.
Visualization: links that take the form of mental pictures rather than words are easier to recall.

How does it work?

Let's say you want to remember to buy cheese, candles, and paper napkins—the only items you still need for your friend's birthday party. A grocery list consisting of only 3 items seems pointless and, moreover, you are likely to lose it. Instead you could link cheese, candles, and napkin in the following funny image: picture your friend wearing a colorful paper napkin tucked into his shirt collar, blowing out 100 candles set on a giant Gouda cheese.

If you spend a few seconds thinking about this image, the chances are you will easily recall it when you are in the store.

DID YOU KNOW: NAME YOUR AUDIENCE When introduced to the 100 people who came to listen to his lecture on memory, Frank Felberbaum managed to memorize 90 of their names (both first and last). He attributed this incredible memory performance to the Link System he used. Frank Felberbaum is one of the world's leading memory experts, and he was also the winner of the Gold Medal at the World Memory Olympics, held in the United Kingdom in 1995.

Practice using the Link System

The following exercises will help you practice creating funny visual images to link random pieces of information and boost your memory of them. You will quickly see how easy and effective it is to use this technique.

12: Bizarre links

Create links for each set of random words listed below. Remember to create associations that are exaggerated and silly to help the objects stick in your mind. For example, if you had to link the words "pedicure" and "lemon pie," you could imagine squeezing lemons with your incredibly lovely feet to prepare the lemon pie. Yes, it's totally bizarre, but memorable! Now it's your turn. Use a separate sheet of paper if you require more space.

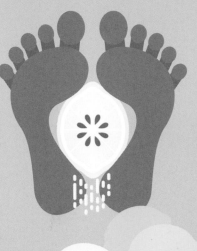

▶ **A:** apple – cow

▶ **B:** pencil – bridge

▶ **C:** phone – grass

▶ **D:** glasses – water

▶ **E:** bag – car – fork

▶ **F:** dog – flower – ruler

▶ **G:** umbrella – scissors – mouse

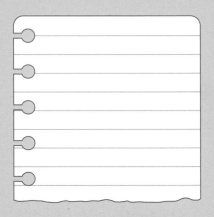

13: Crazy images

The funnier and crazier your visual images, the better. Let's practice visualizing events that are silly and surreal. Create a mental picture of each scene described below. Make sure your images are as detailed as possible. Spend at least 10 seconds on each.

▶ **A:** Marilyn Monroe standing on your sofa wearing a cowboy outfit

▶ **B:** A cockroach smoking a cigar while riding a large motorcycle

▶ **C:** A bearded man wearing only shorts, juggling baby elephants

▶ **D:** A kangaroo sitting in a bathtub filled with marmalade

▶ **E:** A woman with 4 arms playing both a guitar and a trumpet

▶ **F:** A talking lizard helping a group of blue children cross a busy street

▶ **G:** Bruce Lee in swimming trunks in your kitchen chopping carrots with his left hand

▶ **H:** You watering lollipops with a pink fluid on a bright summer's morning

14: Who's ordered what?

Imagine you are a waiter. Use the Link System to memorize the main courses ordered by each person at the table. To associate the food with a person, use exaggerated and surprising images. Picture each link/association in your mind for at least 10 seconds. Add as many details as possible to your images. When you are done, cover up the picture and say out loud three multiplication tables of your choice. Afterward, write down the main courses that you remember next to the people who ordered them.

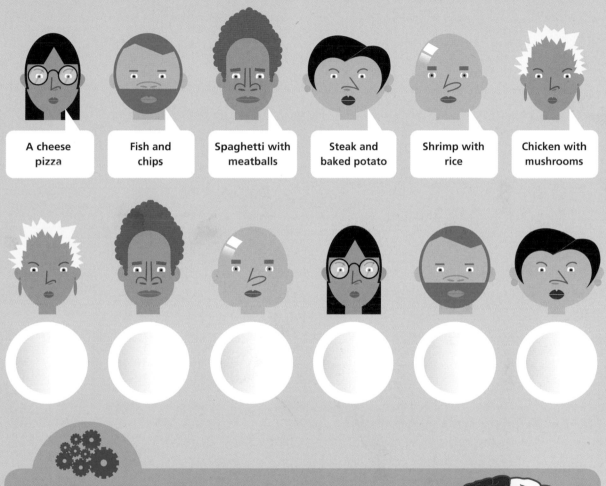

| A cheese pizza | Fish and chips | Spaghetti with meatballs | Steak and baked potato | Shrimp with rice | Chicken with mushrooms |

HOW IT WORKS: BIZARRE IMAGES IN THE BRAIN Which areas of your brain light up when you see (and probably also when you imagine) a bizarre, surprising image (a dog slowly morphing into a watering can, for example)? Neuroimaging studies show that 2 brain regions are active: a network of frontal and temporal brain areas, which are classically associated with the type of deep processing that leads to memory registration, and secondly regions of the brain usually associated with the state of arousal. This explains why such images are remembered so well.

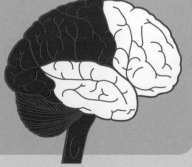

SUPER TECHNIQUE:
The Journey Method

The Journey Method (also known as the method of loci or the memory palace) dates back to Ancient Greek times. It is a very efficient method that combines spatial learning and visualization. The method is useful for memorizing sequences, lists, different points in a speech, material for a test, or even steps to operate a complex machine.

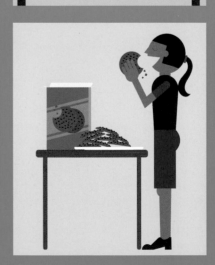
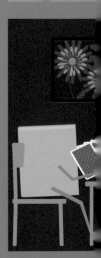

How does it work?

When using the Journey Method, you take a mental walk across a very familiar environment: it can be your house, the route you take to work, or even your own body. Your walk should always start in the same location (for instance, at the front door of your house) and follow the same route (first the dining room, then the kitchen, then the bathroom, the stairs, and so on).

The idea is to create a link between each item on your list and each visited location (or locus). You can merely "leave" an item in a location or more creatively connect the two. What matters is that you take the time to visualize the item in this location and enrich your mental image with as much detail as possible. Later on, when you need to recall the items on your list, you will walk along your mental path and "find" each piece of information where you left it.

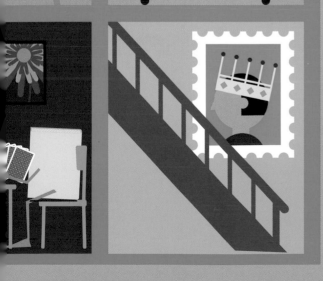

A typical route

Imagine you have a long itinerary of things to do, but don't have a pen to write a list. In the morning you need to go to the post office and then to the library to return books. You are then meeting a friend for lunch. In the afternoon, you have to collect your shirts from the dry cleaners, visit the pet store to buy fish food, and finally buy a few grocery items.

In order to use the Journey Method to memorize this to-do list, first you need to select where your mental walk will take place. Let's say it's a house, like the one illustrated here. This then becomes your "memory palace." There are 6 items on your to-do list, so you will need 6 locations in your memory palace too.

Now you need to link each item on your list to each location. The best way to do this is to use the Link System (see pp.88–89). For instance, you can imagine a poster of a giant "stamp" hanging on the wall of your entrance hall. This will remind you of the post office later on when you mentally enter the house. You can imagine humanlike books sitting at your dining table to remind you of the library, and so on. The more bizarre and surreal the images are, the better your memory for them will be. When you are done, you'll only have to take that journey through your memory palace to locate each to-do item on your itinerary waiting for you in the location you left it earlier.

TOP TIP: CLEAN THE MEMORY PALACE
Many memory champions who use the Journey Method claim that they need to "clean up" their mental locations periodically to avoid cramming them with too much stuff! To get rid of all your links and images, imagine cleaning each location until you can see them as they actually are. In other words, free of any items or bizarre scenes.

Practice using the Journey Method

Complete the following exercises to become familiar with the Journey Method. Thereafter, keep using it as often as possible. Use it to memorize lists that you might refer to at home, school, or work. These could include shopping lists, the periodic table, or even the steps of cardiopulmonary resuscitation (CPR).

15: Build a memory palace

Before using the method, you need to establish which memory palace you are going to use (see p.92 for examples). The key is to pick a location that you are familiar with and which you can navigate with ease.

Once you've chosen your memory palace, take a mental walk through it and pick at least 9 "rooms" (or landmarks) that you know very well.

Next, walk your mind through the same route several times until you know the journey by heart.

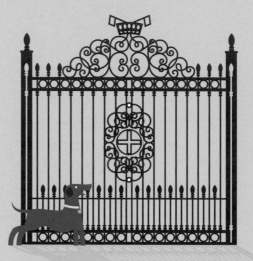

16: Vacation essentials

Use the Journey Method to memorize the vacation shopping list below. Spend 10 seconds placing the items at each location to create a journey filled with vividly detailed, surreal images. For more information on how to build suitable images, refer to the Link System described on page 88. When you are done, cover up the list and, to create a time lag, count backward from 100. Stop after 2 minutes and then write down as many items on the shopping list as you can remember as you work your way through your memory palace.

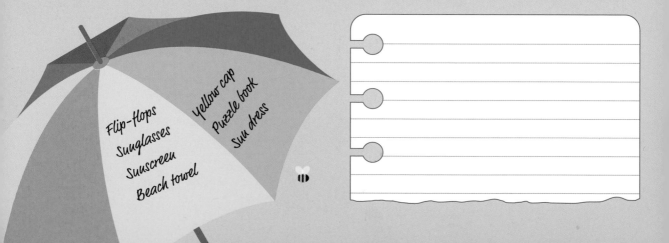

Flip-Flops
Sunglasses
Sunscreen
Beach towel
Yellow cap
Puzzle book
Sun dress

17: Time for dessert

Ready to bake a famous French apple tart? Use the Journey Method to memorize the instructions to prepare a tarte tatin. Visit your memory palace and place/link each step of the instructions to a location. Be imaginative and spend at least 10 seconds at each location.

   Return to the exercise after 10 minutes. Take a mental walk through your memory palace and see how many instructions you can recall. Continue on a separate sheet of paper if necessary.

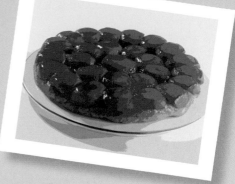

Tarte Tatin

1. Peel and cut apples.
2. Pour sugar into a pot. Add some water and melt it over a low heat and let it caramelize.
3. Add butter to the caramel and stir until it melts.
4. Pour caramel into a dish greased with butter.
5. Quickly place the apples in the dish; pack the slices tightly together.
6. Bake for 40–45 minutes.
7. Leave the dish to cool, then place the crust on top, tucking the edges into the dish.
8. Bake for a further 30 minutes.
9. Once cooled, place a serving dish on top of the tart and flip it over so that the apples are facing up.

HOW IT WORKS: THE JOURNEY METHOD AND PLASTICITY As we age, the brain atrophies. This is due not so much to the loss of brain cells, but their shrinkage and the loss of connection between them. A recent study has shown that brain atrophy can be reversed after 2 months if people learn and recall information daily during this period. Participants in the study used the Journey Method. After 2 months, their memory for lists improved. What's more, scans revealed that the thickness of the cerebral cortex (the outer layer of the brain) had increased in several regions.

Check-out: exercise your imagination for a better memory

It's time to test your memory and the power of your imagination! Calculate your points for each exercise. To boost your score, use the techniques introduced in this chapter, namely the Link System and the Journey Method. You can complete this section over the course of a few days.

18: Time to sketch

How imaginative are you? Add to the doodles below so that each one forms a common object. You have 5 minutes to complete the exercise.

Your score: _____
1 point for each completed doodle

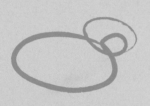
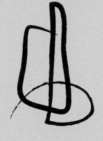
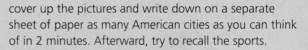
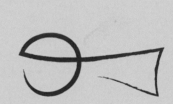

19: A day at the club

Memorize all the sports that are being offered by the new local fitness club so you can inform your friends. Try using the Journey Method. When you are done, cover up the pictures and write down on a separate sheet of paper as many American cities as you can think of in 2 minutes. Afterward, try to recall the sports.

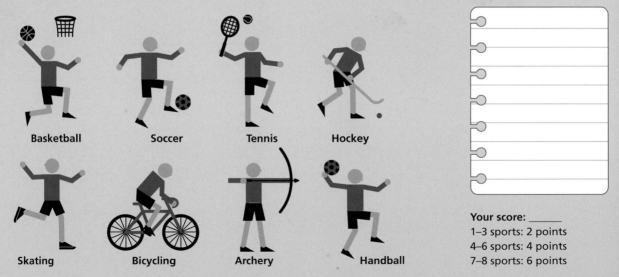

Basketball   Soccer   Tennis   Hockey

Skating   Bicycling   Archery   Handball

Your score: _____
1–3 sports: 2 points
4–6 sports: 4 points
7–8 sports: 6 points

20: Linking game

Find 3 images linking/associating the following items. Each time, try to come up with a powerful image that is memorable. You can describe the images in the space below or draw them on a separate sheet of paper. Complete the exercise in 5 minutes.

Your score: _____
1 link: 1 point
2 links: 2 points
3 links: 3 points

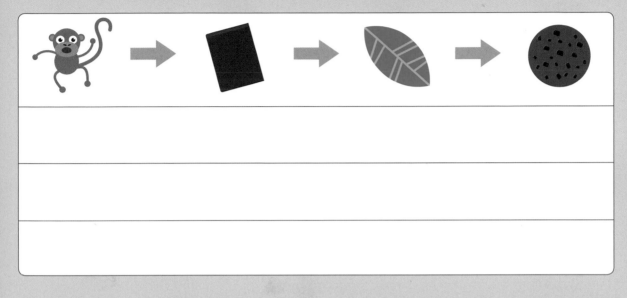

21: United Nations

Use the Journey Method to memorize the 12 members of the European Union as constituted in 1995. You may wish to use the symbols we've provided. Once you are done, close the book. Test your memory after 10 minutes.

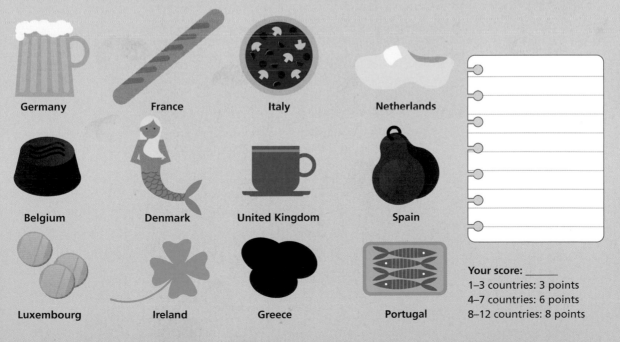

Germany   France   Italy   Netherlands

Belgium   Denmark   United Kingdom   Spain

Luxembourg   Ireland   Greece   Portugal

Your score: _____
1–3 countries: 3 points
4–7 countries: 6 points
8–12 countries: 8 points

22: Linking game (express mode)

On a separate sheet of paper, create a surprising association for each group of items pictured below.

Time yourself and stop after 1 minute. How many links/pictures were you able to create?

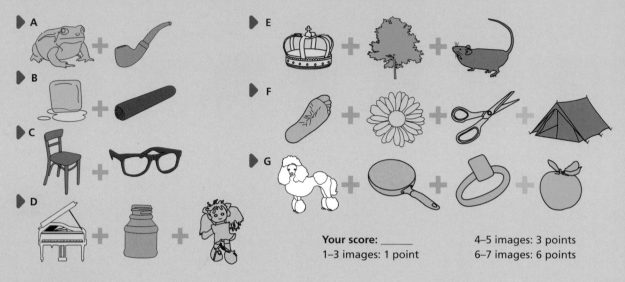

▶ A

▶ B

▶ C

▶ D

▶ E

▶ F

▶ G

Your score: _____
1–3 images: 1 point

4–5 images: 3 points
6–7 images: 6 points

23: Memorize to music

Can you replace the first verse of the well-known children's song below with your new bank account number?

"Twinkle twinkle little star, how I wonder what you are."

Sing the number using the melody that accompanies the line. (If you don't know this song, use one that you do.) Spend a few minutes rehearsing this. When you are done, cover up the number and spend 1 minute trying to solve the riddles in the time lag box. Afterward, recall the account number.

Account number:

2 3 5 6 7 3 0 0 1 5 8

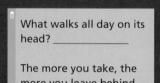

What walks all day on its head? _____

The more you take, the more you leave behind. What is it? _____

Your score: _____
3+ errors: 2 points
2 errors: 4 points
no errors: 6 points

24: Home redecorating

You are about to start work on your kitchen when you realize that you have to run to the store to get the 5 items listed below. Use the Link System to memorize your list. Then cover it up and take 2 minutes to think of as many words as you can starting with the letter V. Afterward, recall your shopping list.

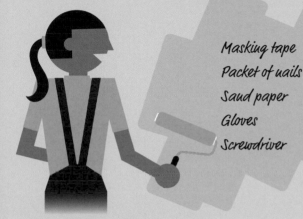

Masking tape
Packet of nails
Sand paper
Gloves
Screwdriver

Your score: _____
1–2 items: 2 points
3–4 items: 3 points
5 items: 4 points

25: The wedding speech

You are the best man at your friend's wedding. You have prepared a speech but prefer not to read it off a sheet of paper. Use the Journey Method to memorize the main parts of the speech. When you are done, solve the math problem. Afterwards, recall out loud as much of the speech as possible (the exact wording does not matter).

$$(120 \times 3) - (25 \times 2) + 54 = \text{\_\_\_\_}$$

$$(80 + 26) + (23 \times 3) - 45 = \text{\_\_\_\_}$$

1. I have known Paul since junior year in high school, and back then he loved chasing girls. Fortunately, he has changed a lot.
2. I was there when Paul and Eva met for the first time. It was not the most romantic situation: Paul was in the car with me when I accidentally hit the bumper of Eva's car at a set of traffic lights!
3. I remember how Paul would always tell me that he would never find a woman who was both smart and caring. Well, he did.
4. I've known Paul and Eva for 5 years and can say that they are perfect for each other.
5. I have never seen them argue except for the time when Paul bought a ladder and they had to carry it all the way home because it did not fit in their car.
May they live happily ever after in their newly painted house (thanks to me!).

Solutions on p.182

Your score: _____
1–2 parts: 2 points
3 parts: 4 points
4–5 parts: 6 points

26: Does it fit in a shoebox?

Visualize each common object below (standard size) and decide whether or not it would fit in an average shoebox. Mark a check or an x beside each item.

Your score: _____
1–4 items: 2 points
5–8 items: 4 points
9–10 items: 6 points

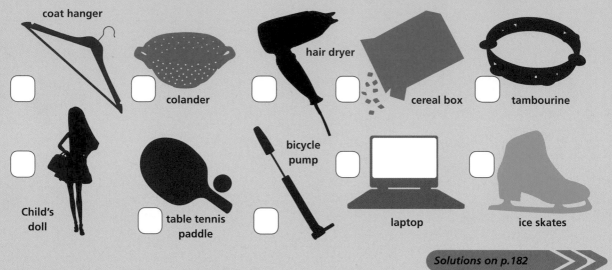

coat hanger

colander

hair dryer

cereal box

tambourine

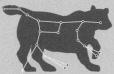

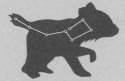

Child's doll

table tennis paddle

bicycle pump

laptop

ice skates

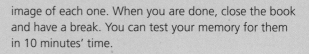

Solutions on p.182

27: Up in the sky

Try to memorize the 6 well-known constellations that are listed below using the Journey Method. Refer to the description of the constellations to create a concrete image of each one. When you are done, close the book and have a break. You can test your memory for them in 10 minutes' time.

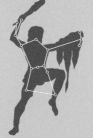

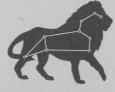

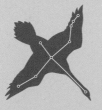

▶ **A: The Great Bear**: its most famous feature is the Big Dipper

▶ **B: The Lesser Bear**: features a smaller dipper and the North Star is located at the end of the Little Dipper's handle

▶ **C: Cassiopeia: or the Queen**, is composed of five very bright stars that form a "W" shape

▶ **D: The Hunter: or Orion**, features 3 bright stars that form a beltlike pattern

▶ **E: The Swan**: one of the largest constellations, forms a crosslike shape

▶ **F: The Lion**: whose head and mane are marked by stars arranged like a reversed question mark

Your score: _____
1–2 constellations: 2 points
3–4 constellations: 4 points
5–6 constellations: 6 points

28: Learn the dance steps

Dancers often rehearse steps mentally when they are outside the dance studio. Let's try the same thing with the dance steps below. Read one step at a time and imagine performing it several times in your head. When you feel ready, stand up and give it a try! Record how many moves you remember to perform correctly.

1. Start, standing up, with both feet together

2. Step to the side with the right foot

3. Step across the right foot with the left foot

4. Step to the side with the right foot

5. Touch the left foot beside the right

6. Then, step back with the left foot

7. Step back with the right foot

8. Step back again with the left foot

9. Touch the right foot beside the left

Your score: _____
1–3 moves: 2 points
4–6 moves: 4 points
7–9 moves: 6 points

29: Surprise gifts

While shopping with your friend, you try to make a mental note of what she seems to like so you can come back later and buy her a surprise present. Use the Link System to memorize the items. When you are done, cover the words and recite the 12 multiplication table. Afterward, write down the items you remember.

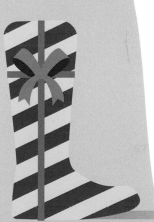

Scarf
Pearl necklace
Bracelet
Pocket mirror
Handbag
Pair of boots

Your score: _____
1–2 items: 2 points
3–4 items: 3 points
5–6 items: 5 points

30: Cube folding

Time for a quick visualization exercise! Let's test your ability to mentally fold and rotate an object. Carefully study the cube template below (left), and decide which of the 4 cubes it would become if you were to fold it.

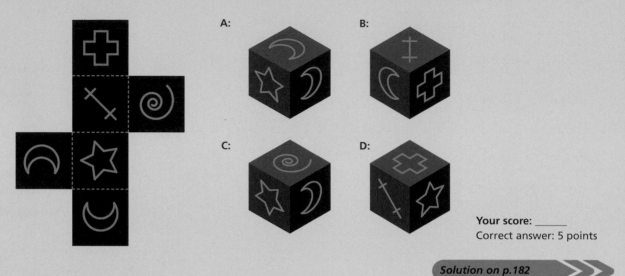

A:

B:

C:

D:

Your score: _____
Correct answer: 5 points

Solution on p.182

31: Red wines

You are applying for a job in a vineyard and need to memorize the different types of red wines and their characteristics. Try using the Journey Method to do this. Use the flavors to come up with a concrete image for each wine. When you are done, cover up the list and take a 10-minute break. Afterward, recall each wine and its description on a separate sheet of paper.

Your score: _____
1–2 wines: 2 points
3–4 wines: 4 points
5–6 wines: 6 points

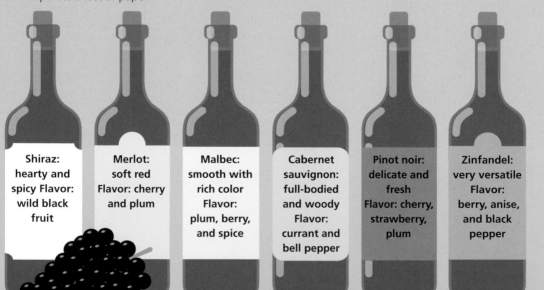

Shiraz: hearty and spicy Flavor: wild black fruit

Merlot: soft red Flavor: cherry and plum

Malbec: smooth with rich color Flavor: plum, berry, and spice

Cabernet sauvignon: full-bodied and woody Flavor: currant and bell pepper

Pinot noir: delicate and fresh Flavor: cherry, strawberry, plum

Zinfandel: very versatile Flavor: berry, anise, and black pepper

32: Connect the 4

Let's test the strength of your associations by assessing how long they last. Take 2 minutes to link/associate the 4 unrelated words below. Visualize your association. Then cover up the words and recite the 4 multiplication table until you reach 64. When you are done, try to recall the 4 words. Then test your memory again after 30 minutes and once more after 1 hour.

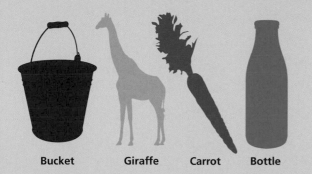

Bucket   Giraffe   Carrot   Bottle

Your score: _____
1–2 words: 1 point
3–4 words: 2 points
30 minutes later:
1–2 words: 2 points
3–4 words: 4 points
1 hour later:
1–2 words: 4 points
3–4 words: 5 points

33: A full schedule

You are a very busy person and have filled every day of the week with an activity. It is getting difficult to keep track of what you're doing on each day. Try using the Journey Method to memorize the sequence of activities. When you are done, cover it up and add up the points you have scored in the check-out so far. Afterward, list the activity you plan to do on each day of the week.

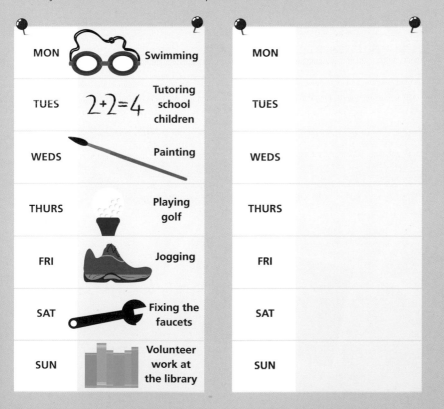

MON	Swimming
TUES	Tutoring school children
WEDS	Painting
THURS	Playing golf
FRI	Jogging
SAT	Fixing the faucets
SUN	Volunteer work at the library

MON	
TUES	
WEDS	
THURS	
FRI	
SAT	
SUN	

Your score: _____
1–2 activities: 1 point
3–5 activities: 3 points
6–7 activities: 5 points

HOW DID YOU DO?
Add up the points you got for each exercise:
your score = (____ x 100) ÷ 93 = ____ %
Are you getting used to the Link System and the Journey Method? Test yourself in a few days' time to see if you've held on to some of the information you memorized in these exercises: keep using the techniques until you master them to experience their full benefits.

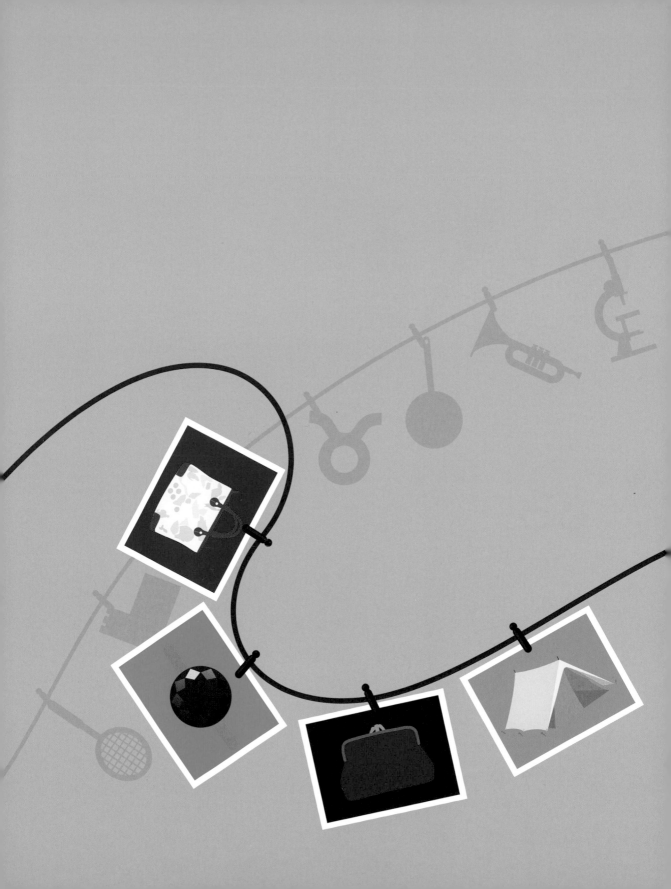

CHAPTER 5

CREATING AN ORDERLY CABINET OF MEMORIES (ORGANIZATION AND MEMORY)

Check-in: how organized is your mind?

You may be wondering what organization has to do with memory. First, the ability to organize information (text, words, pictures) in a meaningful way helps you understand the information better. Second, it creates a system for you to be able to recall the items, which boosts your memory for that information. Before exploring the different ways information can be organized, let's test your natural ability to do this with the following exercises.

1: Accessories

Imagine you are working in a retail store and have been asked to display the accessories below. Can you group the accessories so that you have 3 different categories with 3 items on each shelf? You have 1 minute to do this.

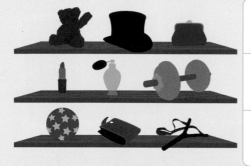

1	
2	
3	

Your score: _____
Found 1 group: 1 point
Found 2 groups: 2 points
Found 3 groups: 3 points

2: Ranking game

Below are pictures of a variety of random objects. Although they are unrelated, can you find 2 ways to rank or order the objects to help you memorize them?

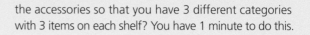

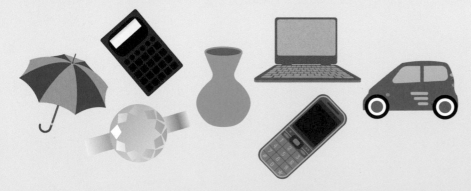

1	
2	

Your score: _____
Found 1 way to order
the objects: 2 points
Found 2 ways to order
the objects: 4 points

3: What's on my kitchen table?

Look at the items on the table with the red tablecloth. Take 1 minute to figure out 3 meaningful groups/categories to put the items into. Then do the same with the items on the table with the blue tablecloth.

Your score: _____
Found 3 groups for table A: 3 points
Found 3 groups for tables A and B (6 groups in total): 6 points

Table A: Table B:

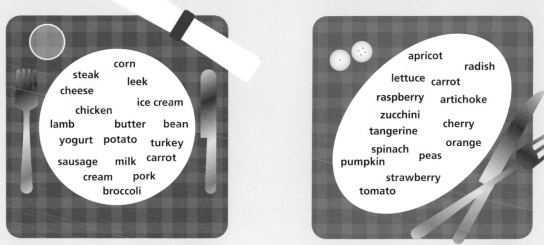

corn
steak   leek
cheese
          ice cream
  chicken
lamb   butter   bean
  yogurt potato   turkey
sausage   milk   carrot
     cream   pork
       broccoli

apricot
              radish
lettuce carrot
raspberry   artichoke
  zucchini
              cherry
 tangerine
              orange
  spinach   peas
pumpkin
        strawberry
  tomato

1	2	3

1	2	3

4: Going fishing

The fish below may look very similar but they actually belong to different species. Take 30 seconds to figure out how many species there are and identify the specific characteristic of each species you find.

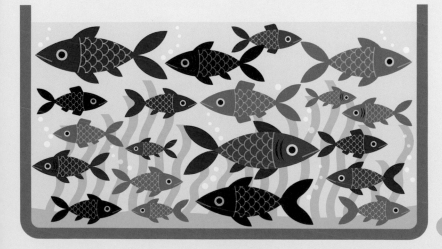

Your score: _____
1 point for identifying each species and its specific characteristic

Solutions on p.183 ≫≫

5: Who are they?

A: A baggage handler at the airport accidentally drops the suitcases belonging to 3 people. Unfortunately, the contents spill out and get mixed up. He has the idea of sorting them according to the profession he can ascribe to each of them. Can you correctly sort the contents and guess the profession of each person?

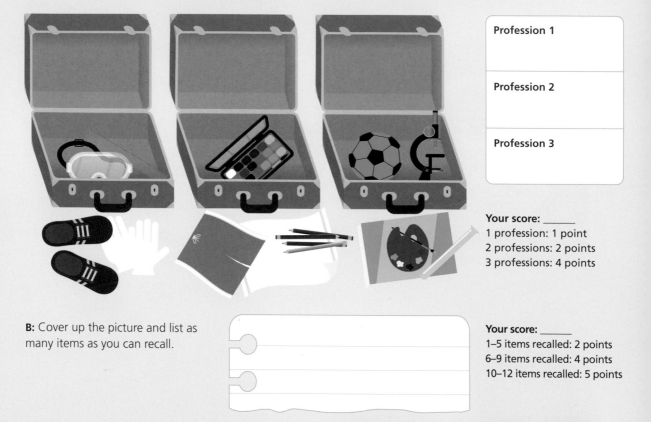

| Profession 1 |
| Profession 2 |
| Profession 3 |

Your score: _____
1 profession: 1 point
2 professions: 2 points
3 professions: 4 points

B: Cover up the picture and list as many items as you can recall.

Your score: _____
1–5 items recalled: 2 points
6–9 items recalled: 4 points
10–12 items recalled: 5 points

6: Sliding puzzle

Take no more than 10 seconds to mentally reorder the squares in the puzzle below so that you create a picture that depicts a famous event in history. Can you name the famous historical event?

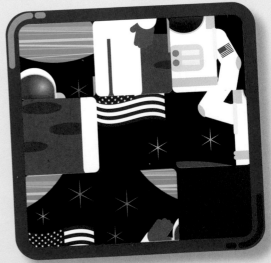

Your score: _____ 2 points for correct answer

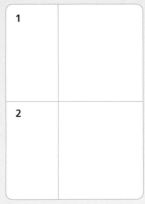

7: Up for grabs

You are participating in a memory recall competition and would like to win first prize. Take 2 minutes to find a way to divide these objects into 2 meaningful groups to help you memorize them. Each group should have the same number of objects.

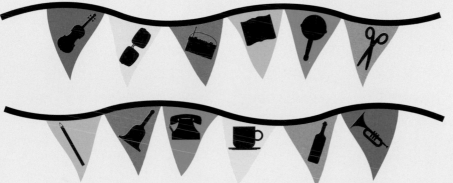

1	
2	

Your score: _____
Identified both groups:
4 points

8: Sorting shapes

Take 30 seconds to figure out the 3 ways to rank/order the shapes below.

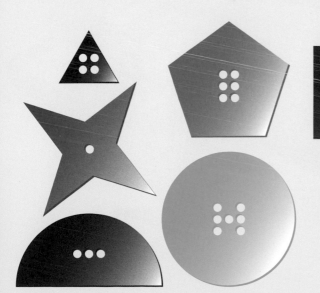

1
2
3

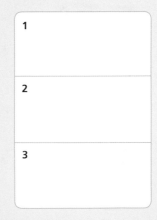

1 0

HOW DID YOU DO?

Time to add up your points. **Your score = (_____ x 100) ÷ 35 = _____ %** Does your score indicate that you have a natural talent for organizing information? How useful is this going to be in your quest for a better memory? Turn to the next page and begin to discover how (and why) organizing the material you want to remember can boost your memory.

Your score: _____
1 ordering system: 1 point
2 ordering systems: 2 points
3 ordering systems: 3 points

Solutions on p.183

Why keeping an orderly mind boosts your memory

If you are looking for a document on your desk, it is usually easier to find if your desk is organized. This is because an organized desk has been tidied up according to rules you have established and a logic that makes sense to you: mail may be stacked by date of arrival, to-do tasks could be in a separate pile, and official papers might be filed away in a specific drawer. So when you need to find something, you know where to look because the categories you used to arrange the contents of the desk act as cues to retrieve specific items.

Organizing information

Memory works in the same way. By organizing the material you want to memorize, you will create groups/categories that will serve as cues for later recall. In addition, the relationships between the items within each category will be strengthened simply because you have established a connection between them. And of course, you cannot organize material without really understanding it, which also helps boost your memory of it.

Let's say you've started a new job and have to learn the names of the different companies you will be dealing with. A long list of company names will be hard to memorize. This is when creating an organized list will come in handy. For example, grouping the companies according to the service they provide can help you form a memory of them. Later on, when you try to recall the company names, you can use these categories as cues to jog your memory. Similar companies will be linked together, too, which increases your chances of remembering them. How about using the same system to memorize the 24 pictures on the next page?

9: What belongs where?

Study the pictures below for 3 minutes and try to identify categories you can group them into (hint: you can form 4 groups). Then cover up the pictures, and to create a time lag, count to 90 in multiples of 3. Afterward, try to recall as many of the pictures as possible.

▶ **A:** List below the categories you identified.

▶ **B:** How many pictures can you remember?

1
2
3
4

Solutions on p.183 ▷▷▷

TOP TIP: YOUR PERSONAL SYSTEM IS THE BEST Many psychological studies have proven that material presented in an organized manner is better remembered than randomly presented material. In addition, creating your own system of organization works better than using one that is given to you. This takes advantage of another memory-boosting effect: we remember better what we come up with ourselves than what we passively receive. So do not hesitate to reorganize any material you need to learn according to a system that makes more sense to you.

Ordering information

Grouping information into meaningful categories is one system of organization that can be used to boost memory. You can also organize information by ordering or ranking it. This can be done by alphabetical order, ascending size, brightness of color, and so on. Use the exercises below to practice using grouping and ranking as a way to improve your memory.

10: Night at the casino

You are at the casino. You need a toilet break and leave your chips with a friend but want to make sure he doesn't gamble any of them in your absence. Take 2 minutes to memorize the chips below. To boost your recall, try ordering them by ascending value. Then cover up the chips and on a separate sheet of paper write down the names of 10 movies you've seen in the last year. Afterward, try to recall all the chips.

11: The mobile zoo

The mobile zoo is visiting your local school. Memorize the different animals the zoo keepers will bring with them, pictured below, so that you can tell the other teachers. How about ranking the animals by size to enhance your recall? When you're done, cover up the animals. To create a time lag, return to exercise 10 and add up the values of all the chips. Afterward, return to this exercise and try to remember all the animals.

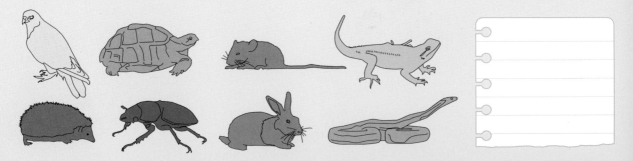

12: Weekend shopping

Here is a list of the things you need to buy over the weekend. To make sure you do not forget any of the items, organize the list based on the 3 stores in which the items can be found. Once you are done, cover up the list and count backward from 150. Stop at 115. Afterward, try to recall all the items on your list.

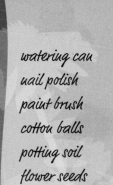

watering can   bandages
nail polish   light switch
paint brush   rake
cotton balls   cough drops
potting soil   masking tape
flower seeds   vitamin pills

DID YOU KNOW: ACRONYMS AND ACROSTICS Acronyms (words that combine the initial letters of a series of words) are famous memory boosters. They organize material in a compressed form, which is easy to memorize. You can use these to remember lists. For instance, the to-do list "go to the **P**ost office, pay **E**lectricity bill, call **A**nna" could become PEA. When acronyms cannot be formed, acrostics can be used. These are memorable sentences or poems in which the letter at the beginning of each word or sentence spells a list of other words. For instance, in music, a well-known acrostic to remember the notes that fall on the lines in ascending order on the treble key is "Every Good Boy Deserves Fudge" (for E, G, B, D, F). You can create acrostics to remember many things, such as the planets in the solar system, the colors of the rainbow, and so on.

SUPER TECHNIQUE:

The Peg System

The Peg System is an efficient way of memorizing random lists of information, such as the 10 most populated countries in the world or the 12 signs of the zodiac. It works by learning a standard set of peg words on which you can hang the information you need to remember. The Link System (see pp.88–89) is used to hang or link information on the pegs.

Create your pegs

First you need to build your pegs. There are different types of pegs: the most common are the rhyming pegs and the alphabetical pegs.

Let's focus for now on the rhyming pegs. For this, you memorize a list of common words, which then become your pegs. You choose words that you can associate with numbers 1 to 10 through rhyme, for example 1 = gun, 2 = shoe, 3 = tree, 4 = door, and so on.

The resulting peg list will be easy to memorize. Remember that you do not have to use numbers. In the alphabetical peg system, letters are used instead to anchor the pegs. In fact, you can use any sequence that you already know by heart.

Once you have learned your peg list, you are ready to memorize any list of items. The peg list only has to be memorized once. Then it can be used over and over again by hanging items you

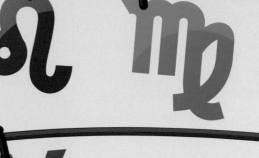

want to memorize on the pegs.
Items are hung on the pegs by using the
Link System (see pp.88–89) so that each item is
visually associated to a peg. For example, if the first
item on your shopping list is milk, you can link it to
the first peg (gun) and imagine a gun firing a jet of
milk. This way, you create a funny and
memorable image that
combines the two.

Let's make it work!

Let's try to use the Peg System to memorize the names of the five most
populated countries in the world: China, India, the US, Indonesia, and Brazil.
You need 5 pegs. Let's say your peg list is as follows: 1 = gun, 2 = shoe,
3 = bee, 4 = door, 5 = dive. Now you need to create strong visual links between
each country and peg. You could imagine 1: a gun firing grains of rice
(China); 2: trying to cross the Ganges River holding your shoes above your
head (India); 3: the American flag with bees instead of stars (US); 4: opening a
door to an archipelago of islands (Indonesia); 5: attending a pool party and
needing a swim to cool off having danced the samba for hours (Brazil). When
you try to recall the names of these countries later on, you will only need to
think of your pegs and you'll instantly remember the vivid images you created.

TOP TIP: THE PEG SYSTEM VS THE JOURNEY METHOD Since both
the Peg System and the Journey Method can be used to memorize lists and
random bits of information, which method should you use? The Peg System
takes more time and effort to learn, but is thought to be more effective. It
may work better than the Journey Method because it doesn't require you
to retrieve items in a sequence. Indeed, you do not need to retrieve your
pegs in order, whereas in the Journey Method you need to visit all the
locations in your memory palace to retrieve the items on your list (see
pp.92–93). So, forgetting a peg will not interfere with the recall of
subsequent information in the same way as forgetting a location would.
To make an informed choice, try both and see which works best for you!

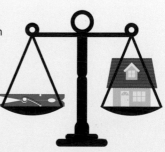

Practice using the Peg System

First you will need to build your list of pegs. Use the step-by-step method described in exercise 13 below. Then practice hanging information on your pegs by completing the other exercises on these two pages. The most demanding part is creating your own list of pegs. You will also need to memorize the pegs; otherwise, you'll have nothing to hang information on!

13: Your personal pegs

▶ **A:** For each numerical peg, from 1 to 10, think of a memorable word (ideally a noun) that rhymes with the number. Take as much time as you need.

▶ **B:** Memorize the words you wrote down for each number. To strengthen the association between the numbers and the words, you can try to:

1 =
2 =
3 =
4 =
5 =
6 =
7 =
8 =
9 =
10 =

1: Visualize the item each word represents. If you wrote down shoe for 2, imagine the shoe: is it a new or old one? What style of shoe is it? What color is it?

2: Draw each item.

3: Practice saying and visualizing the items in a random order (instead of 1 =..., 2 = ..., start at 6 then jump to 4, and so on).

14: Let's go shopping

Memorize the grocery list by linking each item to one of your pegs. Try to create a funny visual association between the two. Then cover up the list and solve the math problems. Afterward, try to recall the items on the list.

$(125 + 41) - (8 \times 2) =$ ___
$(12 \times 6) + (71 + 28) =$ ___
$(23 + 26) + (15 \times 4) =$ ___
$(52 + 20) - (9 \times 8) =$ ___

cookies, beer, ham,
bread, asparagus, eggs,
tea, strawberries

Solution on p.183

15: Top sport

Pictured below are the 10 most popular sports worldwide based on the size of their fan base. Use your pegs to memorize the sports. Cover up the pictures and take a 2-minute break. Afterward, try to recall the sports.

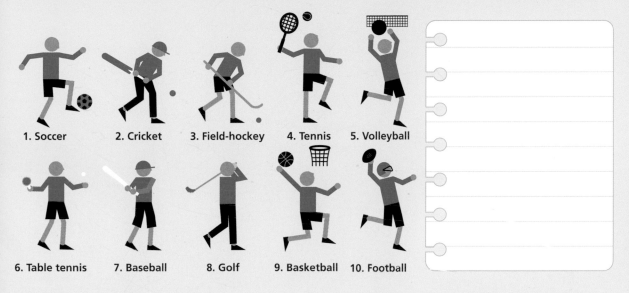

1. Soccer   2. Cricket   3. Field-hockey   4. Tennis   5. Volleyball

6. Table tennis   7. Baseball   8. Golf   9. Basketball   10. Football

16: What to cook tonight?

You have 10 grandchildren who are fussy eaters. It's not easy to remember what everybody dislikes, which makes cooking for family reunions difficult! Use your pegs to memorize the list of foods your grandchildren dislike. Test your memory in 30 minutes' time by writing down the foods below, making sure the list is covered up.

broccoli
mashed potatoes
raw onion
chocolate cake
salmon
cooked carrots
lemon pie
hard-boiled eggs
red peppers
cucumber

HOW IT WORKS: PEG POWER!
The Peg System is a mnemonic that can double your power of recall. You may be wondering whether using the same list of pegs over and again would create interference and induce forgetting. This is not the case. Studies show that using pegs boosts recall and this effect is maintained despite repeatedly using the same pegs.

SUPER TECHNIQUE:
Create Mind Webs

A Mind Web organizes ideas or facts in a visual way. Information is represented in the form of a central idea connected to a network of other related ideas. This is inspired by how information is organized in the brain, namely, in networks of interconnected concepts. Mind Webs can be used to learn, understand, and memorize material ranging from the contents of a lecture to the details of a business strategy or personal plan.

ORGANIZE WEDDING DAY

How does a Mind Web work?

A Mind Web is not linear—it represents information in a visual, radial way. A typical Mind Web starts with a key word or image representing the central idea of the information you are dealing with. Associated ideas, grouped by themes, are then attached to the central idea: they literally branch out from it. Less important ideas are attached to these associated themes via smaller branches, and ideas of even lesser importance sprawl out as offshoots from the smaller branches.

The creation of a Mind Web forces you to engage with the material on a detailed level, thereby increasing your understanding of it. Such deep processing combined with the visual representation of the material explains why Mind Webs act as memory boosters. In addition to their role in learning, Mind Webs can be used for problem solving, preparing presentations, or planning an event.

Invitations

Select stores

Gift registry

Using the Mind Web technique

Let's say you are helping a friend to organize her wedding day. There are so many things to consider that neither of you knows where to begin. In this instance, building a Mind Web can be the perfect solution to make sure you approach the task with a sound strategy and you don't forget anything.

As you can see, the main idea—"organize wedding day"—is placed at the center. In this example, the main parts of the event have been separated into four categories or branches: guests, bride and groom, food, and location. From each of these sprout related minor branches. For instance, from the major branch "guests" sprout smaller ones such as "invitations," "gift registry," and so on. From a minor branch sprout further offshoots, such as "select stores." Once complete, the Mind Web shows at a glance everything that needs to be done to organize the wedding. Since it is visual, it boosts the organizers' memories for what they need to do.

DID YOU KNOW: THE FIRST MIND WEB The use of Mind Webs can be traced back to the 3rd century BC, when a Greek philosopher used one to illustrate a complex concept developed by Aristotle. However, it was not until the 1950s that the link between this kind of mental mapping and effective human learning was discovered (seminal work was carried out by Dr. Allan Collins and Ross Quillian in the 1960s). Modern Mind Webs have been popularized by psychology author Tony Buzan, who has coined the term "mindmap" to describe this tool. Nowadays you can even find software that helps you build Mind Webs.

Practice using Mind Webs

Use the exercise below to create a Mind Web. The web is partly drawn to give you a head start. Begin with the main themes and then start branching out. There is no limit to the number of branches and sub-branches you can create. If the space provided on the page isn't enough then use a separate sheet of paper. Take all the time you need to complete the exercise.

17: Long vacation

You are thinking of going on a month-long trip to Bolivia and Brazil. You start looking on the Internet for more information and find a useful site: *www.travelindependent.info/america-south.htm*. Read the webpage and then draw a Mind Web to see whether you can visually organize the information that is most relevant to you. To get you started, we've already put down the central idea and 5 main branches. Complete the Mind Web. Test your memory 30 minutes after completion by writing down the information you can remember on a separate sheet of paper.

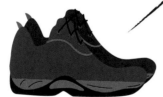

Clothes

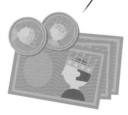

Money

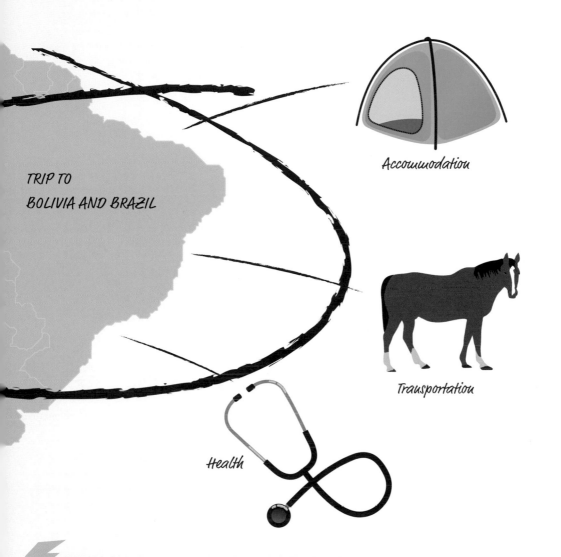

TRIP TO
BOLIVIA AND BRAZIL

Accommodation

Transportation

Health

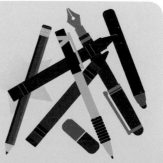

TOP TIP: BE CREATIVE When you are creating a Mind Web, do not hesitate to erase and redraw. Use different colored pens and vary the thickness and length of lines. Include as many images as possible (small motifs representing ideas) and limit the amount of written information. It doesn't have to be a work of art, but something that triggers a memory. The more visual details you have in the Mind Web, the better. Include anything that seems relevant to your central idea. Above all, be creative! Creative maps will boost your power of recall the most because they are visually striking and also because you spend more time building them.

Check-out: exercise organizing information into solid memories

How good have you become at organizing information for a better memory? Do these exercises to discover the answer. Try to use the Peg System, a Mind Web, or a grouping system when recommended. Record your points for each exercise. You can complete the section over the course of a few days.

18: Bird watching

Below are 6 birds common to the US or UK. Take 1 minute to memorize their names. (Try putting them into 2 groups to boost your memory of them.) Then cover them up and move on to exercise 19. Afterward, write down the correct name under each bird.

Your score: _____
1–2 birds: 2 points
3–4 birds: 4 points
5–6 birds: 6 points

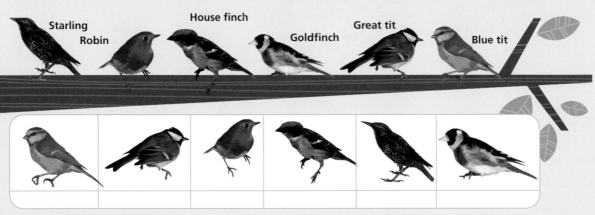

Starling
Robin
House finch
Goldfinch
Great tit
Blue tit

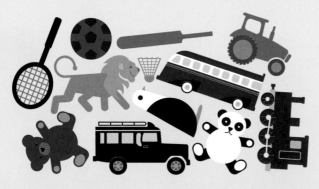

19: A trove of toys

Can you memorize all the toys pictured below? To boost your memory, group the toys into meaningful categories.

When you're done, cover up the toys and, on a separate piece of paper, list as many green-colored fruits as you can think of in 2 minutes. Afterward, try to recall the toys. (Do not forget to return to exercise 18.)

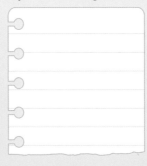

Your score: _____
1–4 toys: 3 points
5–8 toys: 6 points
9–12 toys: 9 points

20: The coldest places on Earth

Below is a list of the 10 coldest locations in the world. Try using your pegs to memorize them. When you are done, cover up the names and complete the math problems. Then try to recall the locations in descending order starting from the coldest nation.

$(12 \times 6) - (4 + \underline{\quad}) = 56$

$(5 \times 8) + (7 - \underline{\quad}) = 42$

$(60 \div 4) + (26 - \underline{\quad}) = 29$

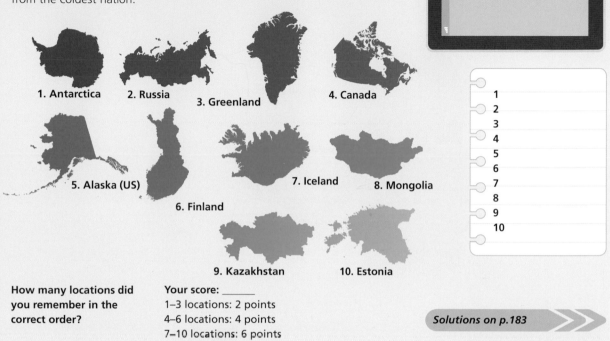

1. Antarctica
2. Russia
3. Greenland
4. Canada
5. Alaska (US)
6. Finland
7. Iceland
8. Mongolia
9. Kazakhstan
10. Estonia

1
2
3
4
5
6
7
8
9
10

How many locations did you remember in the correct order?

Your score: _____

1–3 locations: 2 points
4–6 locations: 4 points
7–10 locations: 6 points

Solutions on p.183

21: Ring fingers

Can you memorize all the rings on the woman's fingers? Work out the grouping system to help you here. Once you're done, cover up the rings and solve the time-lag problem. Afterward, circle the rings you recognize in the display below.

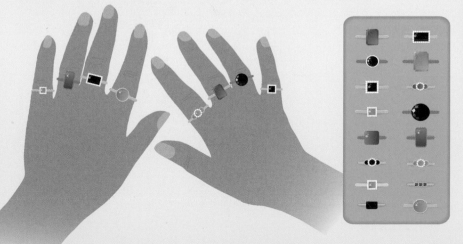

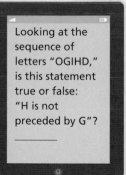

Looking at the sequence of letters "OGIHD," is this statement true or false: "H is not preceded by G"?

_____

Your score: _____

1–3 rings: 2 points
4–6 rings: 4 points
7–8 rings: 6 points

22: Journalism school

So you want to become a journalist. Do you know the 6 main questions you should answer when filing a report? The questions are:

Try using your pegs to memorize these questions. If your first peg is "gun," then you could visualize a scene in which someone in a mask is stealing your gun, prompting you to ask: "Who stole the gun?" When you are done, cover up the list and recite the 7 multiplication table. Afterward, try to recall the checklist questions.

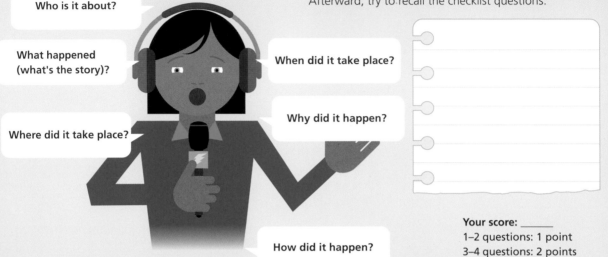

Who is it about?

What happened (what's the story)?

When did it take place?

Why did it happen?

Where did it take place?

How did it happen?

Your score: _____
1–2 questions: 1 point
3–4 questions: 2 points
5–6 questions: 3 points

23: Beautiful bouquet

Imagine you are a florist. A customer calls to order a bouquet but your pen runs out of ink and you can't write down the order. Can you memorize the flowers he wants? How about organizing them by color to improve your recall? When you are done, cover up the picture and write down on a separate sheet of paper as many types of tea as you can think of in 1 minute. Afterward, write down below as many types of flowers as you can remember from the order.

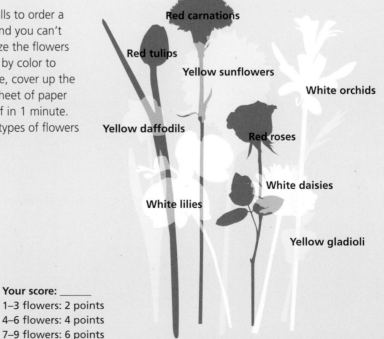

Red carnations

Red tulips

Yellow sunflowers

White orchids

Yellow daffodils

Red roses

White daisies

White lilies

Yellow gladioli

Your score: _____
1–3 flowers: 2 points
4–6 flowers: 4 points
7–9 flowers: 6 points

24: To the rescue

Your neighbor is an elderly lady for whom you often run errands. She called you this morning with a list of things for you to do. To make sure you remember all the tasks, use the Peg System (see pp.114–115) to memorize the to-do list. When you are done, cover up the list and take a 2-minute break. Afterward, see how many tasks you can recall from the list.

take prescription to the pharmacy
mow her lawn
order special socks online
check her bank statement
buy milk and flour for her
renew her newspaper subscription
show her how to send an email

Your score: _____
1–3 tasks: 2 points
4–5 tasks: 4 points
6–7 tasks: 6 points

25: Cloud gazer

Try to memorize as many cloud names as you can in the chart below. Use the shape of the clouds as well as their elevation as organization principles to help boost your recall. Then cover up the cloud names and complete the math problems below. Afterward, write down the correct name of each cloud in the blank chart.

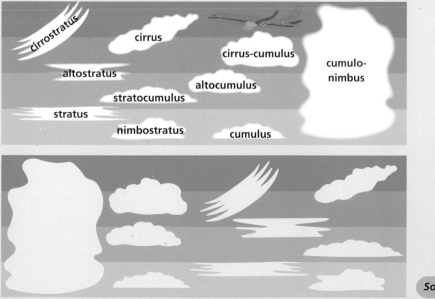

cirrostratus
cirrus
cirrus-cumulus
altostratus
altocumulus
cumulo-nimbus
stratocumulus
stratus
nimbostratus
cumulus

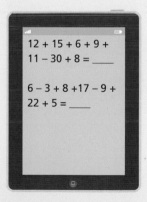

12 + 15 + 6 + 9 + 11 − 30 + 8 = ____

6 − 3 + 8 +17 − 9 + 22 + 5 = ____

Your score: _____
1–3 cloud names: 2 points
4–6 cloud names: 4 points
7–10 cloud names: 6 points

Solutions on p.184

26: The great outdoors

The last time you went on a camping trip, you forgot several essential items. To make sure this doesn't happen this time round, you decide to memorize the most important items you'll need. Try using your pegs to do this. Then cover up the list and answer the question in the time lag box. Afterward, write down as many items as you can remember.

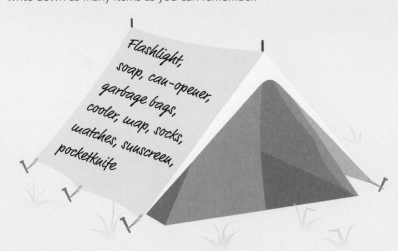

Flashlight, soap, can-opener, garbage bags, cooler, map, socks, matches, sunscreen, pocketknife

List 4 favorite books from your childhood
1:
2:
3:
4:

Your score: _____
1–3 items: 2 points
4–6 items: 4 points
7–10 items: 6 points

27: Entertaining James

Your nephew James, who is 5 years old, is visiting you and your family next week. You need to keep him and your son busy and are looking for things to do with them. Using your nearest city as a model, plan for the week by drawing a Mind Web on a separate sheet of paper. Think of the things that are available in your area. Include any different kinds of entertainment you can think of (such as arts and crafts, outdoor activities, museums, playgrounds) and don't forget to add suitable places for lunches and snacks.

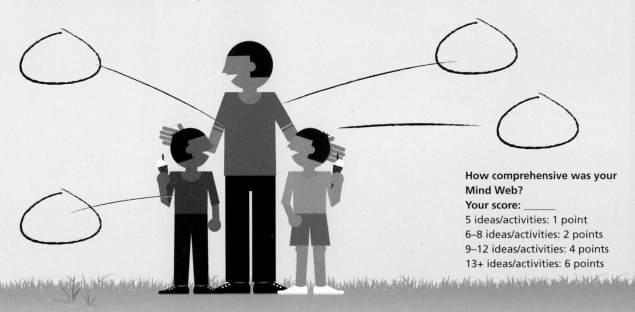

How comprehensive was your Mind Web?
Your score: _____
5 ideas/activities: 1 point
6–8 ideas/activities: 2 points
9–12 ideas/activities: 4 points
13+ ideas/activities: 6 points

28: Decathlon

Do you know the order of the events in a decathlon? As the name indicates, it includes 10 sporting disciplines that are spread over 2 days. Can you memorize what happens on each day? You may want to use the Peg System here. When you are done, complete the math problems. Afterward, try to remember the 10 events of a decathlon, in the correct order if possible.

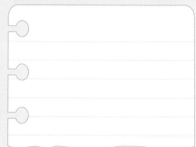

$(230 - 90) + (15 \times 4)$
$= \underline{\hspace{1cm}}$

$(124 - 12) + (8 \times 6) - (45 + 9) = \underline{\hspace{1cm}}$

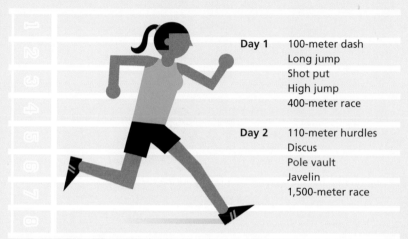

Day 1	100-meter dash
	Long jump
	Shot put
	High jump
	400-meter race
Day 2	110-meter hurdles
	Discus
	Pole vault
	Javelin
	1,500-meter race

Solutions on p.184

Your score: _____
1–4 events: 2 points
5–8 events: 4 points
9–10 events: 6 points
Add 2 points extra if you remembered the events in the correct order.

29: Fixing the house

You need to repair parts of your house before you can put it up for sale. The picture below shows the 8 most urgent things that need fixing. To aid memorization, try organizing the repairs from top to bottom. Then cover up the picture and take 2 minutes to think of as many boys' names as you can beginning with B. Afterward, try to recall the 8 parts you need to repair.

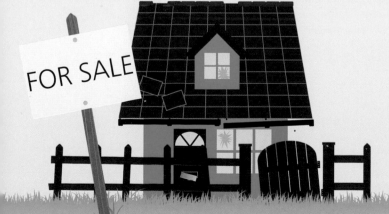

Your score: _____
1–3 parts: 2 points
4–6 parts: 4 points
7+ parts: 6 points

30: Time to limber up

It's difficult to do an exercise routine while referring to a fitness manual. Why not memorize the program in advance? Here is a sequence of exercises that is great for building body strength. To memorize the exercises, try ordering them starting at the legs and then move upward. When you are ready, cover up the exercises and count backward starting from 65. Afterward, see how many exercises you can remember.

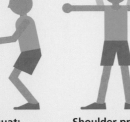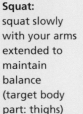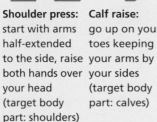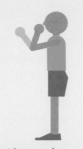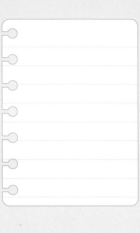

Squat: squat slowly with your arms extended to maintain balance (target body part: thighs)

Shoulder press: start with arms half-extended to the side, raise both hands over your head (target body part: shoulders)

Calf raise: go up on your toes keeping your arms by your sides (target body part: calves)

Bicep curl: bend arms at 90° in front of you, curl upper arms toward shoulders (target body part: biceps)

Leg extension: hold your hips and raise one leg to the side and then alternate (target body part: buttocks)

Your score: _____
1–2 exersises: 3 points
3–5 exercises: 6 points

31: Caring for your car

Any car requires a variety of regular checks to ensure that it is safe to drive. Use the Peg System to memorize the essential maintenance checks. Once you're done, say the alphabet out loud missing out alternate letters. Afterward, cover up the information in the top box and fill in the blank spaces below.

Your score: _____
1–2 words: 2 points
3–4 words: 4 points
5–6 words: 6 points

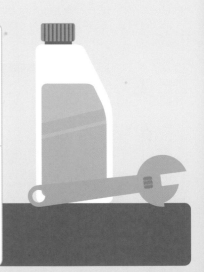

Maintaining a car
• Check fluids: brake fluid, transmission fluid, power steering fluid, oil, washer fluid, engine coolant (antifreeze)
• Tires: check pressure, balancing, rotation, wheel alignment, wear
• Inspect or replace windshield wipers, air and fuel filters, oil, spark plugs, belts
• Check all lights

Maintaining a car
• Check fluids: brake fluid, _____, power steering fluid, oil, _____, engine coolant
• Tires: check _____, balancing, rotation, wheel alignment, _____
• Inspect or replace _____, air and fuel filters, _____, spark plugs, belts
• Check all lights

32: Vegetable garden

You have decided to plant the following fruits and vegetables in your new garden. Try using your pegs to memorize them. When you are done, cover up the garden and on a separate piece of paper list as many breeds of dogs as you can think of in 2 minutes. Afterward, test your memory of the produce.

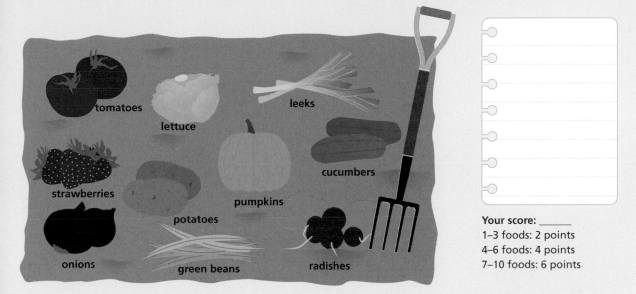

Your score: _____
1–3 foods: 2 points
4–6 foods: 4 points
7–10 foods: 6 points

33: Lost in the forest

Can you memorize the shapes of these different leaves and the names of the trees they belong to? To boost your recall, try putting the leaves into meaningful groups (such as those with pointy ends, those that are prickly, and so on). When you're ready, cover the leaves and recite the 6 multiplication table backward from 60. Afterward, draw the leaves and write down the names of the tree they belong to on a separate piece of paper.

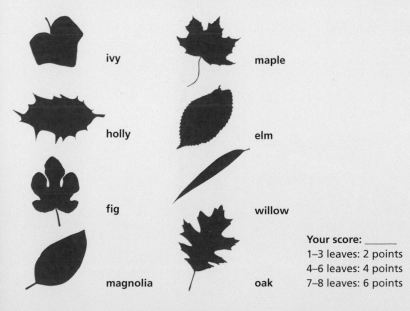

Your score: _____
1–3 leaves: 2 points
4–6 leaves: 4 points
7–8 leaves: 6 points

1 0

HOW DID YOU DO?
Time to add up your points.
Your score = (_____ x 100) ÷ 98 = _____ %
You are working hard: congratulations! By now, you should have memorized your pegs and be ready to use them when required. Try drawing Mind Webs whenever you need to organize and memorize a lot of information. Of course, do not hesitate to review the techniques in the previous chapters so that you can decide which best suits your needs.

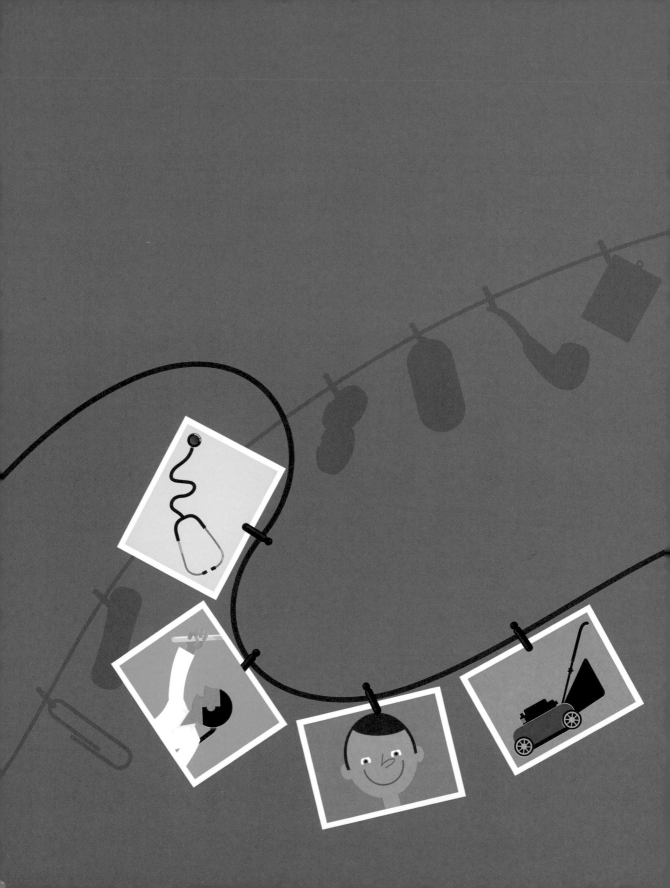

CHAPTER 6

REMEMBERING NAMES AND FACES

Check-in: how well do you remember names and faces?

Before learning how to boost your memory for names and faces, let's test your current ability. Once more, we've added an unrelated time-lag task for some of the exercises. Write down your score as you go along and add up your points at the end.

1: Meeting the board

Below are the names of the 8 members you want to speak to at the next board meeting. Take 1 minute to memorize their names. Then cover them up and count backward from 30. Afterward, see how many names you can remember.

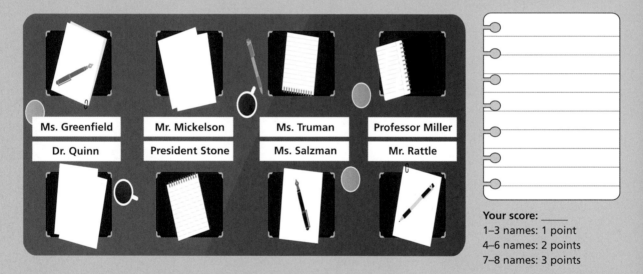

| Ms. Greenfield | Mr. Mickelson | Ms. Truman | Professor Miller |
| Dr. Quinn | President Stone | Ms. Salzman | Mr. Rattle |

Your score: _____
1–3 names: 1 point
4–6 names: 2 points
7–8 names: 3 points

2: New bank workers

Study the faces of these 5 new bank employees. After 30 seconds, cover them up and recite the 7 multiplication table backward from 70. Afterward, circle the 5 employees who match the ones below among the three rows of faces on the next page.

Your score: _____
1–2 faces: 1 point
3–4 faces: 2 points
5 faces: 3 points

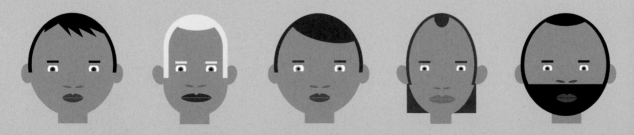

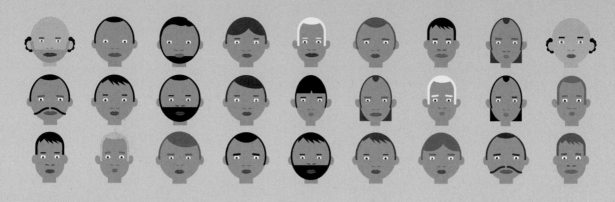

3: Name the faces

Take 1 minute to memorize the names and faces on the right. Once you're done, cover them up and take a 2-minute break. Afterward, write down the correct names under the faces below.

Ruth Raugh   James Weisman   Nancy Kemna   Matthew Steele

Your score:_____
1 point for each name recalled under the correct face

4: Observing faces

Take 2 minutes to look closely at the 4 faces below. Try to memorize as much as you can about them. Now cover up the faces and, to create a time lag, spell out 10 words that each consist of 6 letters. Afterward, see how many of the questions on the right you can answer correctly.

A: What is Mr. A's hair color?

B: Is Ms. B wearing glasses?

C: Does Mr. C have thin lips?

D: Does Ms D. have long hair?

E: Does Mr A. have thick eyebrows?

F: Does Mr C. have a flat or pointy nose?

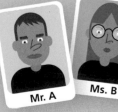
Mr. A

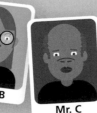
Ms. B

Mr. C

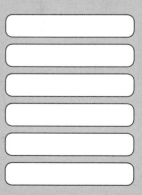
Ms. D

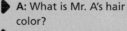
Solutions on p.184

Your score: _____
1–2 correct answers: 1 point
3–4 correct answers: 2 points
5–6 correct answers: 3 points

5: Back to the bank

Without referring back to exercise 2 on page 132, can you still identify the 5 new bank employees from the array of faces below? (They are all now wearing a pair of glasses to make things a little more difficult.) Circle the correct faces.

6: Pairing up

You are introduced to 3 couples at a dinner party. Take 30 seconds to memorize the names and faces of each couple. Then cover them up and recite the alphabet backward starting from the letter J. Afterward, fill in the correct names under the picture of each couple.

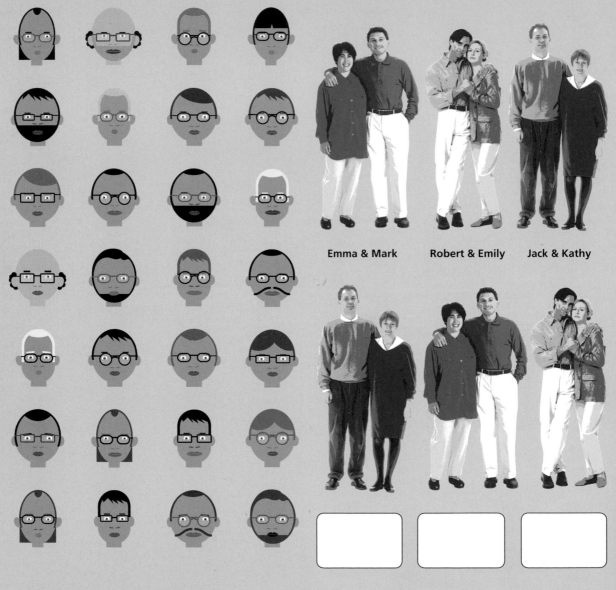

Emma & Mark   Robert & Emily   Jack & Kathy

Your score: _____
1–2 faces: 1 point
3–4 faces: 2 points
5 faces: 3 points

Your score: _____
1 point for each couple
identified correctly

7: Star-studded cast

You read a review of a Hollywood blockbuster starring 5 leading male actors. Take a few minutes to memorize the 5 names. Then cover them up and think of the names of 10 female actresses. Afterward, see how many actors' names you can remember.

TOM HANKS MATT DAMON

JOHNNY DEPP   BRAD PITT

LEONARDO DICAPRIO

Your score: _____
1–2 names: 1 point
3–4 names: 2 points
5 names: 3 points

8: On a day trip

Here are 5 children you have to look after during a trip to the aquarium. Take 1 minute to memorize their names and faces so that you can find them if they wander off. Then cover them up and solve the math problems. Afterward, recall their names and draw an arrow to the correct faces.

26 + 51 + 32 + 64 = _____
43 + 31 + 36 − 20 = _____
34 + 45 + 7 − 21 = _____
32 + 12 − 30 + 11 = _____

Elsie   **Daniel**   **Alice**   **Robert**   **Ashley**

Solutions on p.184

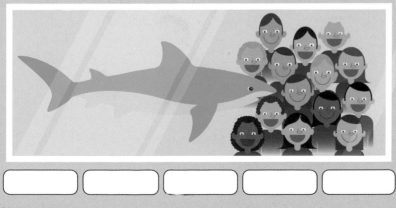

Your score: _____
1–3 faces only: 1 point
4–5 faces only: 2 points

1–3 faces + names: 3 points
4–5 faces + names: 4 points

1 0

HOW DID YOU DO?
Time to add up your points.
Your score: _____ ÷ **26 points**
(_____ **x 100) =** _____ **%**
Are you pleasantly surprised? Or do you feel your memory for names and faces needs to improve? Whatever the case, read on to understand why names are so hard to memorize. There are a few tricks that you can use to boost your memory for them, too. The next pages will help you master these.

SUPER TECHNIQUE:
The 3-Step Memory Booster

We all forget names at times, whatever our age. Names seem to have a habit of going in one ear and out the other. Remembering names is not impossible, though. Here are two simple and efficient methods to help you.

Two simple methods

The first method is repetition. Repeating someone's name when you first meet that person will increase your chances of remembering it later. The simplest way to do this is to use the name as you talk to the person. For example, "Rebecca, I was wondering whether…?"; "What do you think about …, Rebecca"; and so on. The other method is the 3-Step Memory Booster. The goal of this technique is to associate the name to a concrete visual object, which will then become your cue to remember the name.

How does the 3-Step Memory Booster work?

This method makes use of association and visualization in the same way as the Link System (see pp.88–89).
• The first step is to give the name a concrete meaning. Some names, especially surnames, such as Miller or Greenfield, already have a meaning. However, although most names don't offer an immediate meaning, they can still remind you of something concrete. For instance, Watson may remind you of Dr Watson in Sherlock Holmes. If you listen to the sound of the name, you can also hear "what son?".
• The second step is to observe the face of the person whose name you are trying to remember. Pay close attention to the individual features. Are the eyebrows thick and bushy? Is the nose big? Are there any moles? Select a facial feature that is striking to you.
• The third step is to link the name and face into a single image. Imagine the object the name reminds you of attached to the striking facial feature you have selected. So "Mr. Shelley" might have a shell stuck in his bushy eyebrows. Although silly, the image is memorable. This final step strengthens the link between face and name. However, the first two steps can be enough to boost your memory for the name.

Let's try it!

You are introduced to Mrs. Chisholm. To begin with, make sure you've got the name right. Ask her to repeat it, and maybe even spell it for you.

Step 1 What does the name remind you of? Maybe you know somebody else with the same name? Maybe the sound of the name makes you think of a "chisel" or a combination of "cheese" and "elm"? Let's say you pick "chisel."

Step 2 Study Mrs. Chisholm's face. You need to focus on the individual features rather than the face as a whole. The way Mrs. Chisholm ties her hair reveals a large forehead. She also has a mole on her chin. Pick either of these as your striking feature.

Step 3 Now combine the name and face in a memorable image using the Link System. Picture a chisel on her forehead, or perhaps an image of a white chisel on a black flag, which is sticking out of her mole. This is indeed ridiculous, but it is also why you will remember her name.

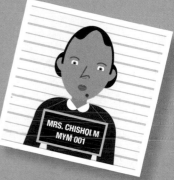

DID YOU KNOW: THE POWER OF THE 3-STEP MEMORY BOOSTER! Are you thinking that the 3-Step Memory Booster is far too complicated, time consuming, and frivolous? First, trust your brain: associations, links, and images come to mind very quickly. Second, note that the mere fact of adding meaning to names (step 1) can boost your memory for them. In one study, a group of people whose average age was 43 were trained for 6 hours over 3 weeks to give more meaning to new names they encountered by using step 1 of the 3-Step Memory Booster. As a result, their memory for names increased and the effect was still present 3 months later. So, yes, it is worth the effort, even if you do not feel like creating silly images every time you meet someone new.

Practice using the 3-Step Memory Booster

These exercises will help you practice the different steps involved in the 3-Step Memory Booster. You will be asked to give first and last names more meaning, observe faces closely, and, finally, associate names and faces to boost your powers of recall. Remember to be creative when it comes to links and associations.

9: New colleagues

Here are the names and faces of 4 new work colleagues. Use the 3-Step Memory Booster to memorize the names and the faces they belong to. For each name, write down what it reminds you of, then select a striking facial feature, and form an image that combines the two. When you are done, cover up the names and, to create a time lag, starting at 51 count down in 3s. Afterward, write down the correct name beside each face.

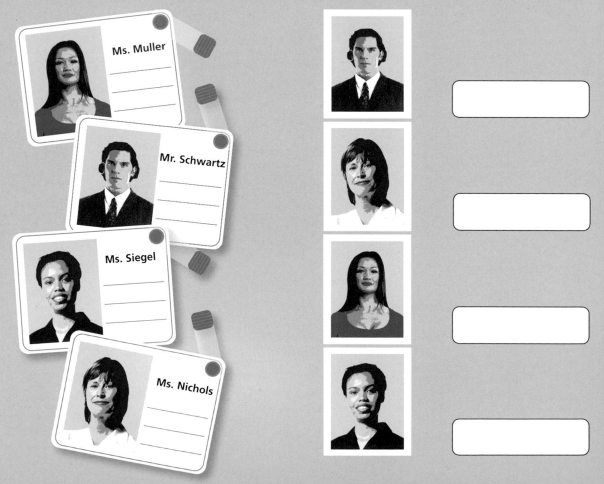

Ms. Muller

Mr. Schwartz

Ms. Siegel

Ms. Nichols

10: Meaningless names?

Let's try to give the names below some concrete meaning. For each name below, write down whether you know someone with the same name (a friend, a celebrity, a work colleague), and then write down what the name reminds you of, in other words, what comes to mind when you read it or say it out loud.

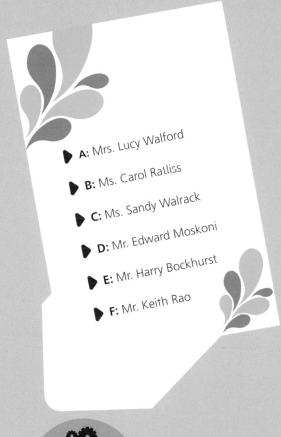

▶ **A:** Mrs. Lucy Walford

▶ **B:** Ms. Carol Ratliss

▶ **C:** Ms. Sandy Walrack

▶ **D:** Mr. Edward Moskoni

▶ **E:** Mr. Harry Bockhurst

▶ **F:** Mr. Keith Rao

HOW IT WORKS: YOUR EYES SEE THE SUM OF ITS PARTS When you encounter a new face, you rarely focus on the individual features. Instead, your brain naturally identifies the relationships between the different features and then processes the configuration of the whole face. In fact, it's what helps you recognize a face and differentiate it from others. There is a simple way to demonstrate this. Take a moment to study the two faces on the right. Can you see any differences between them?

Now turn the book upside down and take another look. Can you now see a difference?

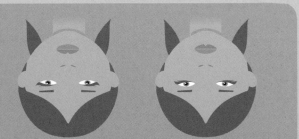

Why was it harder to see the down-turned mouth and eyes of the right-hand face when it was upside down? It's because seeing it upside down disrupted your ability to process the configuration of the face.

Check-out: exercise your memory for names and faces

Now that you're familiar with the 3-Step Memory Booster, let's test your memory for names and faces again. When the exercise asks you to memorize a name, use only step 1 of the method and try to give more meaning to the name to boost recall. When a face is also shown, study it carefully and try to follow the other two steps of the method. You can complete this section over a few days.

11: The new batch

Imagine you're a teacher. Here are 4 new students who are joining your class this year. Take a few minutes to memorize their faces so that you can recognize them later today. Then cover up the faces and, to create a time lag, recite the 3 multiplication table up to 60. Afterward, circle the faces of your students in the group below.

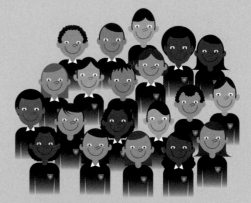

Your score: _____
1 point for each face identified

12: Influential women

Listed below are a few of the most influential women of the 20th century. Take 2 minutes to memorize their names. Then cover them up and recite the 7 multiplication table out loud until you reach 105. Afterward, try to recall the women's names.

- **Susan B. Anthony** (American civil rights movement leader who fought for women's rights)
- **Dorothy Hodgkin** (awarded Nobel Prize in Chemistry for her work on the structure of both penicillin and insulin)
- **Mother Teresa** (humanitarian and advocate for the poor and helpless in India)
- **Indira Gandhi** (first female prime minister of India, who served for three consecutive terms)
- **Rosa Parks** (African-American civil rights activist)

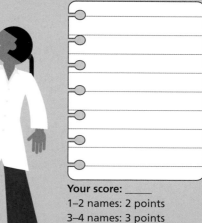

Your score: _____
1–2 names: 2 points
3–4 names: 3 points
5 names: 4 points

13: Postcards aplenty

Over the summer you received many postcards. Can you memorize the names of the people who sent you these? After 2 minutes, cover them up and, starting at 52, count down by 4s. Afterward, try to recall the names of the people who sent you a card.

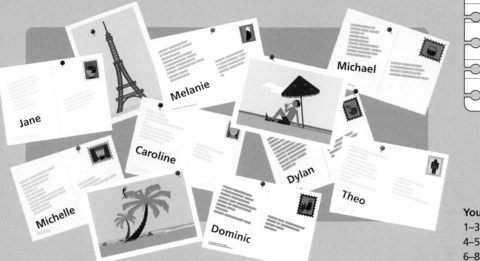

Jane

Melanie

Michael

Caroline

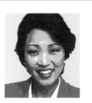

Dylan

Theo

Michelle

Dominic

Your score: _____
1–3 names: 2 points
4–5 names: 3 points
6–8 names: 4 points

14: Meet the teachers

Below are the names and photographs of 6 new teachers at your son's school, as well as the subjects they teach. Take all the time you need to memorize them using the 3-Step Memory Booster. Then cover up the names and faces, and take 2 minutes to remember 2 of your own favorite teachers at school. Write down on a separate sheet of paper the reasons why you liked them. Afterward, answer the questions below.

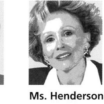

Ms. Walker
English

Mrs. Reed
Math

Ms. Henderson
Geography

Ms. Griffin
Biology

Ms. Crawford
Physical education

Mr. Palmer
History

▶ **A:** Does Ms. Henderson wear earrings?

▶ **B:** What does Ms. Griffin teach?

▶ **C:** Who is the new math teacher?

▶ **D:** Does Mr. Palmer have facial hair?

▶ **E:** Does Ms. Walker wear glasses?

▶ **F:** Who is the new physical education teacher?

Solutions on p.184

Your score: _____
1–2 correct answers: 2 points
3–4 correct answers: 3 points
5–6 correct answers: 4 points

15: Friends of a friend

Your friend introduces you to his friends. Take 1 minute to memorize their names and faces. Then cover them up and solve the time-lag problem. Afterward, write down the names in the answer boxes with an arrow pointing to the correct faces in the picture.

Rebecca

Nathan

Tommy

Tanya

Jessica

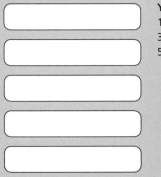

Complete the analogy: sponge is to porous, as rubber is to
a) massive b) wet c) elastic d) dull
_____

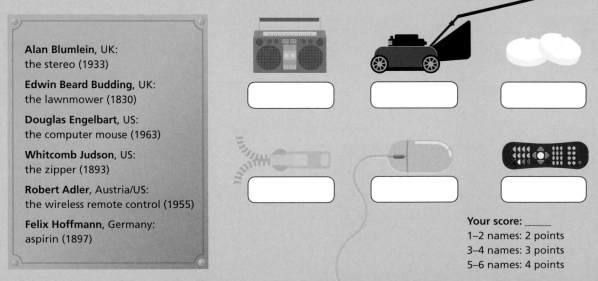

Your score: _____
1–2 names: 2 points
3–4 names: 3 points
5 names: 4 points

16: Who's the inventor?

Do you know the names of the people who invented many of the common objects we use today? We've listed a few below. Take 2 minutes to memorize their names and what they invented. Then cover up the information, and take a 5-minute break. Afterward, write down the name of the inventor under each invention illustrated below.

Alan Blumlein, UK:
the stereo (1933)

Edwin Beard Budding, UK:
the lawnmower (1830)

Douglas Engelbart, US:
the computer mouse (1963)

Whitcomb Judson, US:
the zipper (1893)

Robert Adler, Austria/US:
the wireless remote control (1955)

Felix Hoffmann, Germany:
aspirin (1897)

Your score: _____
1–2 names: 2 points
3–4 names: 3 points
5–6 names: 4 points

17: Business relations

4 people handed you their business cards at the last trade fair. Each card includes a photograph of the person. Take a few minutes to memorize the names using the 3-Step Memory Booster. Then cover up the business cards and complete the math problems in the time-lag box. Afterward, write down the correct names on the business cards below.

18: Too many docs!

Can you memorize the names of the doctors below and what they specialize in? Take as much time as you need, then cover them up,and, on a separate sheet of paper, list the names of the memory techniques you have learned so far in this book. When you're done, write down the correct doctor's name beside each specialism.

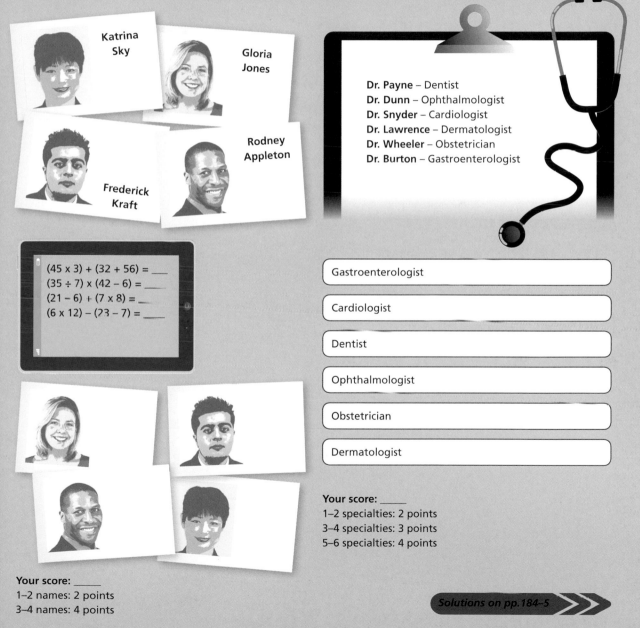

Katrina Sky

Gloria Jones

Rodney Appleton

Frederick Kraft

Dr. Payne – Dentist
Dr. Dunn – Ophthalmologist
Dr. Snyder – Cardiologist
Dr. Lawrence – Dermatologist
Dr. Wheeler – Obstetrician
Dr. Burton – Gastroenterologist

$(45 \times 3) + (32 + 56) = $ ___
$(35 \div 7) \times (42 - 6) = $ ___
$(21 - 6) + (7 \times 8) = $ ___
$(6 \times 12) - (23 - 7) = $ ___

Gastroenterologist

Cardiologist

Dentist

Ophthalmologist

Obstetrician

Dermatologist

Your score: _____
1–2 specialties: 2 points
3–4 specialties: 3 points
5–6 specialties: 4 points

Your score: _____
1–2 names: 2 points
3–4 names: 4 points

Solutions on pp.184–5

19: On first-name terms

Below are the first names of the distinguished guests you would like to meet at the next art show. Memorize the names in 2 minutes, then cover them up and solve the time-lag problem. Afterward, draw a circle around the names of the people you want to talk to in the lower list of names.

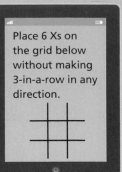

Place 6 Xs on the grid below without making 3-in-a-row in any direction.

Douglas	Fiona	Patrick	Heidi
Colin	Olivia	Richard	Rachel

Rachel   Vanessa   Eleanor   Gabriel
Dustin   Patrick   Benjamin   Douglas
Pamela   Fiona   Olivia   Adam
Heidi   Colin   Philip   Ella
Oscar   Patricia   Bianca   Richard

Your score: _____
1–3 names: 2 points
4–6 names: 3 points
7–8 names: 4 points

20: Party time!

As you chat with the party hostess, 4 guests arrive and the hostess introduces them to you. Can you memorize their names and faces? Once you're done, cover up the names and faces and complete the math problems. Afterward, write down the correct name under each face.

$67 + 45 - 6 =$ ____
$34 + 4 - 8 =$ ____
$23 - 7 + 26 =$ ____
$424 - 234 =$ ____

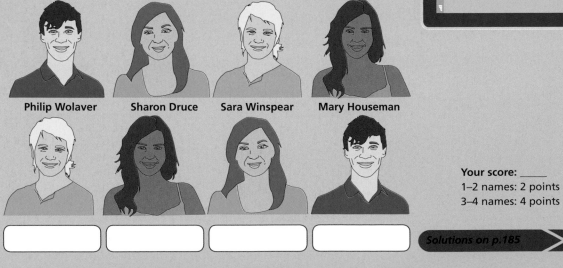

Philip Wolaver   **Sharon Druce**   **Sara Winspear**   **Mary Houseman**

Your score: _____
1–2 names: 2 points
3–4 names: 4 points

Solutions on p.185

21: Who's playing?

Imagine you've seen a poster advertising a concert in which 8 famous singers are performing. Can you memorize their names? Once you're done, cover up the poster, and on a separate sheet of paper, take 2 minutes to list as many words as you can think of beginning with the letter U. Afterward, try to recall the singers' names.

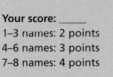

Your score: _____
1–3 names: 2 points
4–6 names: 3 points
7–8 names: 4 points

Elton John
Prince
Celine Dion
Eric Clapton
Annie Lennox
George Michael
Whitney Houston
Alicia Keys

22: The philanthropic six

On the right are the names of the 6 volunteers who will help you organize a charity event. Try using the 3-Step Memory Booster to memorize their names. When you're done, cover up the names and faces, and take a 5-minute break. Afterward, write down the names you remember under the correct faces below.

Mr. Frazier

Ms. Burke

Mr. Vargas

Ms. Pearson

Ms. Chambers

Mr. Osborne

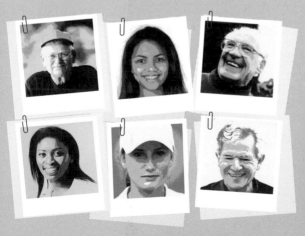

Your score: _____
1–2 names: 2 points
3–4 names: 3 points
5–6 names: 4 points

1 0

HOW DID YOU DO?
Time to add up your points:
Your score = (_____ x 100) ÷ 48 points = _____ %
Compare this with your check-in score. Have you improved? Try using the 3-Step Memory Booster the next time you meet someone. You'll be surprised at how well you remember the person's name later on. The more you use the method, the easier it will become, and soon it will feel like second nature!

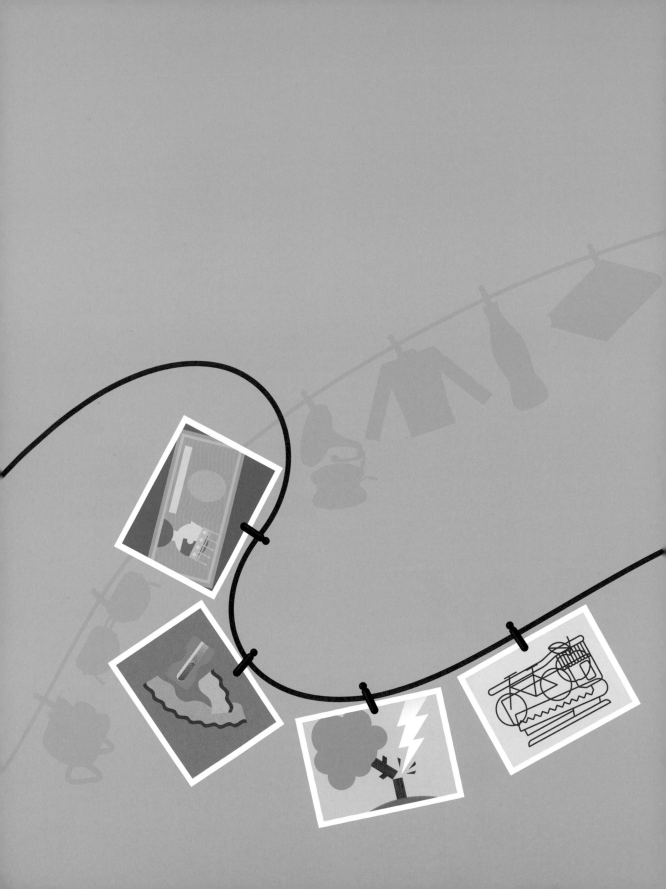

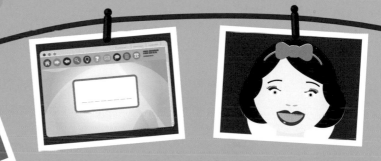

CHAPTER 7
REMEMBERING NUMBERS

Check-in: do you have a head for storing numbers?

For most people, it's a challenge to memorize numbers, be it a phone number or a PIN. Fortunately, a few simple techniques and a willingness to learn can help you become more proficient at memorizing numerical information. Before discussing these techniques, let's assess your current memory for numbers.

1: Window shopping

Can you memorize the prices of the following items of clothing? Study each price tag for 10 seconds, then cover them up and, on a separate sheet of paper, list as many girls' names beginning with A as you can think of in 1 minute. This will create a time lag. Afterward, recall the prices of the 3 items.

2: Momentous years

Here are the dates of 3 historical events. Pick one you don't know already and memorize it. When you are done, move on to the next exercise. Afterward, return to this exercise and recall the event and the year it happened.

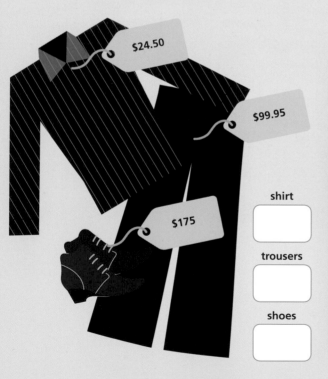

$24.50

$99.95

$175

shirt

trousers

shoes

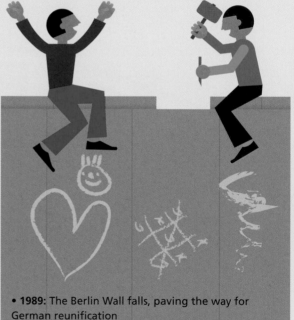

- **1989:** The Berlin Wall falls, paving the way for German reunification
- **1982:** the first music album is released on CD
- **1994:** Nelson Mandela is elected president of South Africa, marking the end of Apartheid.

Your score: ____
1 price: 1 point
2 prices: 2 points
3 prices: 3 points

Your score: ____
Event and year recalled:
3 points

3: Driving too much?

You are about to go on a 6-month trip abroad and reluctantly decide to leave your car with a friend. When your friend drives you to the airport, you think it might be prudent to memorize the reading on the odometer so that you can figure out how much he drives the car in your absence. When you are done, cover it up and take a 2-minute break. Then recall your odometer reading. Afterward, return to the previous exercise.

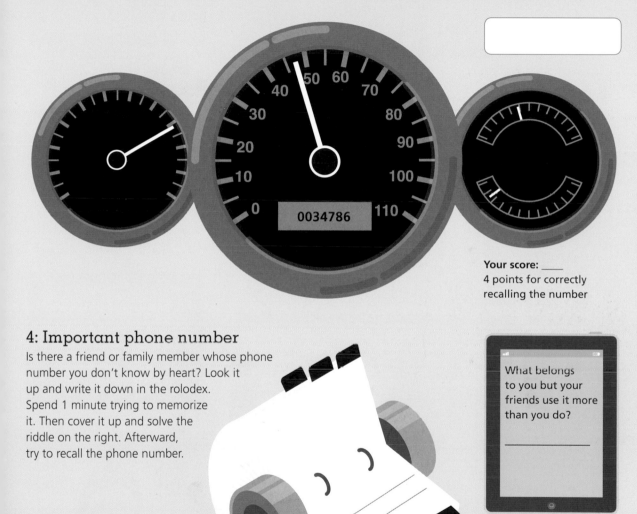

0034786

Your score: _____
4 points for correctly recalling the number

4: Important phone number

Is there a friend or family member whose phone number you don't know by heart? Look it up and write it down in the rolodex. Spend 1 minute trying to memorize it. Then cover it up and solve the riddle on the right. Afterward, try to recall the phone number.

What belongs to you but your friends use it more than you do?

_____

Your score: _____
3+ errors: 1 point
2 errors: 2 points
1 error: 4 points
no errors: 6 points

Solution on p.185

5: Code to enter the site

You have registered for an online service and have been provided with the following access code: **12254930**. Take 30 seconds to memorize it. Then cover it up and solve the riddle on the right. Afterward, recall the code.

A basket contains 5 apples. How can you divide it among 5 children so that each has 1 apple and 1 apple stays in the basket?

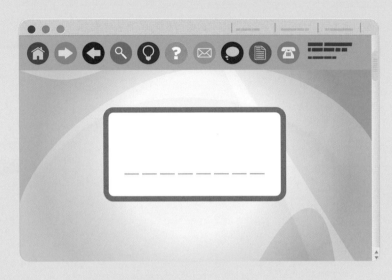

— — — — — — — —

Your score: _____
3+ errors: 1 point
2 errors: 2 points
1 error: 4 points
no errors: 6 points

6: Age is just a number

Take 1 minute to memorize the birth years of the following people. Then cover up the dates and find your way in the maze. Afterward, write down the correct birth year under each person.

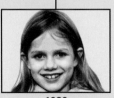

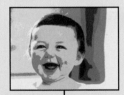

1956

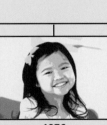

1967

1976

1989

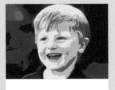

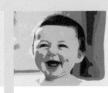

Your score: _____
2 points for each year recalled correctly

7: Knitwear for Christmas

You're knitting sweaters for your 3 nephews this Christmas. Can you memorize their sizes? Take 2 minutes to study the measurements, then cover them up and solve the time-lag problem below. Afterward, recall each set of sizes.

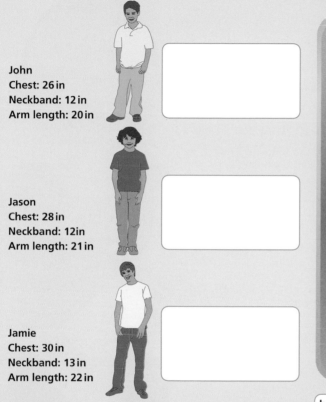

John
Chest: 26 in
Neckband: 12 in
Arm length: 20 in

Jason
Chest: 28 in
Neckband: 12 in
Arm length: 21 in

Jamie
Chest: 30 in
Neckband: 13 in
Arm length: 22 in

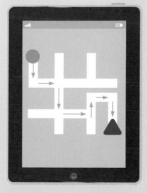

How many left and right turns do you need to take to go from the circle to the triangle? (You're not allowed to rotate the book!)

Your score: ____
1 set of sizes: 1 point
2 sets of sizes: 3 points
3 sets of sizes: 6 points

Solutions on p.185

8: Tight security!

For security reasons, the entry codes to the main building at work and the garage are changed regularly. Can you memorize the 2 new codes? When you are done, cover them up and take a 2-minute break. Afterward, try to recall the 2 entry codes.

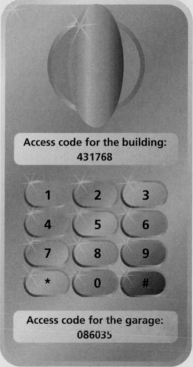

Access code for the building:
431768

1	2	3
4	5	6
7	8	9
*	0	#

Access code for the garage:
086035

building

garage

Your score: ____
1 code: 3 points
2 codes: 6 points

1 0

HOW DID YOU DO?
Add up the points you got for each exercise.
Your score = (____ x 100) ÷ 42 = ____ %
Did you have a hard time trying to memorize and recall all those digits? Or was it not as bad as you thought it would be once you applied yourself? In the next pages, you will be introduced to a few techniques that can help you boost your memory for numbers.

The beauty of chunking

The reason numbers are difficult to recall is because they are abstract concepts. They do not stick in your memory as readily as words or pictures, both of which you can usually attach a meaning to. However, chunking (or grouping) individual digits into larger units is an easy way to boost your memory for them.

Grouping long numbers

Can you memorize the following number inside 30 seconds: 3 4 1 9 9 8 7 4 7? Of course it would be much easier to write the number down than to attempt to cram it inside your head in the short space of time. OK, let's try grouping the number into three units instead: 341 998 747. You now have only three numbers to memorize instead of nine digits. If you repeat these three units out loud several times, your verbal short-term memory (see p.34) is likely to remember the number later on.

Finding meaningful groups

Memorizing numbers becomes even easier when you can attach meaning to them. How is that possible? Well, let's try to find some kind of meaning in what initially seems to have none. The number above can be chunked differently: 34 1998 747. Now, "34" may have been your age when you had your first child, "1998" may be the year you moved into a new house, and "747" may remind you of the most popular airplane in Boeing's fleet. With these associations, the number would now be much easier to memorize and a lot harder to forget!

Of course, in many instances you won't be able to find such personal meanings in numbers. You will then have to be creative and imaginative. To get you started, here is a list of number-related information you may know well enough to use as meaningful chunks:

• Birth dates (of friends and family members, for example)
• Addresses (of places you go to often, for example)
• Historical dates (you learned at school, for example)
• Autobiographical dates (the date you were married, for example)
• Your Social Security number
• The number on the jersey of your favorite sports player
• Famous numbers such as 007 (the fictional British secret service agent), Route 66 (the famous US highway), 3.14 (pi), and so on.

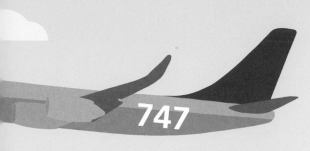

747

9: Trip to Beijing

You are organizing a trip to China, and frequently have to phone the travel agency in Beijing. The phone number is: **008610198253**. Use the chunking method to memorize this number. Try to recall the phone number in 10 minutes' time.

10: A slice of pi

It's perhaps one of the most widely recognized numbers in the world, but how much of it do you know? How about trying to memorize the first 10 digits of this infinite number: **3.141592653**. Once again, use the chunking method to help you. Then cover it up and solve the riddle below. Afterward, recall the number.

What is black when you buy it, red when you use it, and gray when you throw it away?

_____

Solutions on p.185

1998

FOR SALE

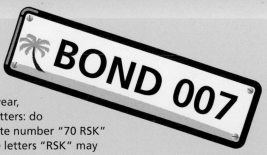

BOND 007

TOP TIP: REMEMBER YOUR LICENCE PLATE NUMBER

Do you have a hard time recalling your licence plate number? Use chunking. Look at your plate number and try to find a chunk of digits or letters that make sense to you: do the digits form a number you know (a year, a memorable date, a special number)? How about the letters: do they remind you of a word? For example, the licence plate number "70 RSK" may remind you of the age of a close friend (70) and the letters "RSK" may remind you of the word "risk." Or, better still, you may combine both in a sentence such as "At the age of 70 it's riskier to go skiing!"

SUPER TECHNIQUE:

The Number-Association System

Here is another method to transform an abstract number into something more memorable: convert it into a picture. This way you can take advantage of the superiority of images in memory (see pp.82–83). There are at least three ways to do this using the Number-Association System.

What is the Number-Association System?

This is a mnemonic system in which numbers are converted into concrete objects, making them easier to visualize. You can do this by associating each number with:

• an object whose name **rhymes** with the number. For example, zero = snow, one = bun, two = shoe, and so on.

• an object whose **shape** looks like the written number. For example, zero = hole, 1 = candle, 2 = swan, and so on.

• an object whose **meaning** is associated with the number. It is up to you which method you choose to use.

Creating meaning

Let's focus on the third method (finding meaning). Here are objects to which each number could be matched:

0 = an empty glass or a black hole (represents nothingness)
1 = the sun (there is only one in our solar system)
2 = twins or eyes (we all have two eyes)
3 = a tricycle (it has three wheels) or a trident (it has three prongs)
4 = a lucky clover (it has four leaves)
5 = a hand (it has five fingers) or a foot (it has five toes)
6 = a fly (it has six legs)
7 = Snow White (because of the seven dwarfs)
8 = a spider (it has eight legs)
9 = a heavily pregnant woman (nine months of pregnancy)

Once you have a list of number-image associations, you need to learn it by heart. Then you are ready to memorize any number. To do so, you need to convert each number into its corresponding object and imagine the objects interacting in a striking visual scenario.

How does it work?

Let's say you have been given a new Personal Identification Number (PIN) for your credit card—7542—and you need to memorize it. First, convert each digit into an object: 7 = Snow White, 5 = hand, 4 = lucky clover, and 2 = twins. Now put together your visual scenario: Snow White is handing you a lucky clover before the twins can snatch it away. Add any details that make the image more striking and therefore more memorable (see pp.84–85): Snow White's hand is white and delicate, the leaf is a bright green color, and so on. Chances are you will now recall your new PIN very easily.

DID YOU KNOW: THE MAJOR SYSTEM This mnemonic works by converting numbers into memorable words. First you need to learn how to convert numbers into consonant sounds. For instance, 1 = d or t (because these letters have only one down stroke), 2 = n (two down strokes), 3 = m (three down strokes), 4 = r (last letter of the word four), and so on. Then the sounds of these letters are transformed into words by adding vowels. For instance, the number 314 could be translated into the word **MeTeoR**, and the number 11 into **ToaD**. The conversion from number to word is phonetic, so it is the consonant sounds that matter, not the spelling.

Practice using the Number-Association System

To use the Number-Association System, you need to build a list of number-image associations that works for you. Start by creating your list and then practice using your number-images to memorize birth dates and PINs.

11: From digits to images

▶ **A:** Transform digits 0 to 9 into visual objects. Create your own set of images using one of the 3 systems described on pp.154–155: rhyme, shape, or meaning. Doodle on a separate sheet of paper if it helps you come up with suitable ideas.

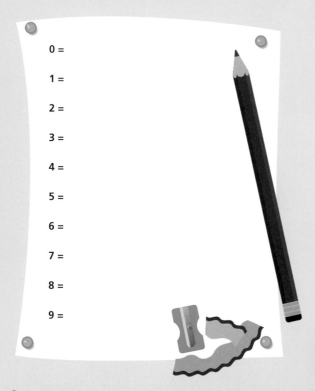

0 =

1 =

2 =

3 =

4 =

5 =

6 =

7 =

8 =

9 =

▶ **B:** Now memorize your list. Test your memory for your list over several intervals. Recall the list by saying it out loud, writing it down, drawing or visualizing the objects. If there's an object you can never remember, then change it. Perhaps it's not the best association for you.

12: Birth years

Use your number-images to memorize the birth years of 3 people you work with. If you happen to work from home, then use the years below:

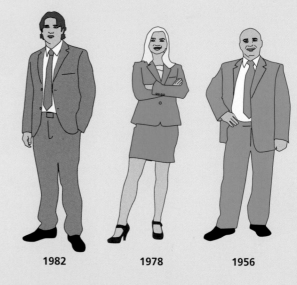

1982   1978   1956

Once you have inserted your number-images into 3 vivid mental scenarios, cover up the years and solve the problem below. Afterward, try to recall your scenarios and in doing so, the 3 years.

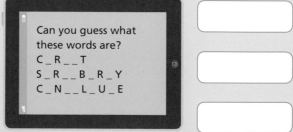

Can you guess what these words are?
C _ R _ _ T
S _ R _ _ B _ R _ Y
C _ N _ _ L _ U _ E

13: Safe delivery

Imagine you are a secret agent and have to deliver 2 briefcases containing sensitive documents. For added security, each lock has a different code; all the codes are shown below. Use the Number-Association System to memorize these codes. When you are done, cover up the numbers and solve the riddle in the time-lag box. Afterward, try to recall the 4 codes.

Q: At night they come without being fetched, and by day they are lost without being stolen. What are they?

_____

A: Briefcase 1

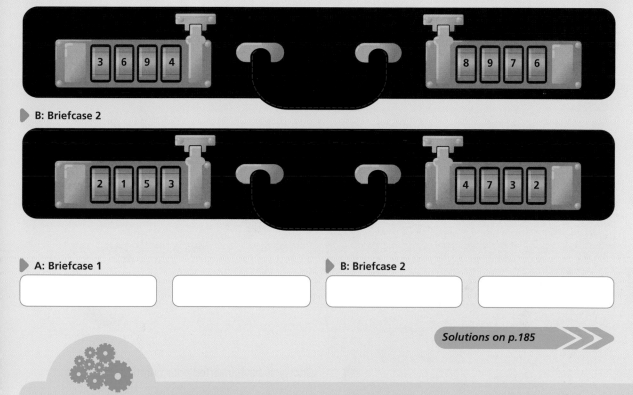

B: Briefcase 2

A: Briefcase 1

B: Briefcase 2

Solutions on p.185

HOW IT WORKS: THE MENTAL DIVIDE When people in a left–right reading culture think of numbers, they automatically think in terms of a number line, with smaller numbers on the left and larger numbers on the right. How do we know this? In a computerized exercise, in which subjects had to press a key to the left of the keyboard when certain numbers appeared on the screen and a key to the right when other numbers appeared, the results showed that people reacted much faster when they had to press the left key for small numbers and the right key for larger numbers. This experiment reveals how the brain spatially maps numerical information in order of ascendancy, depending on the direction our eyes follow while we are reading.

Check-out: exercise your memory for numbers

Now that you are familiar with the techniques, let's assess your memory for numbers once again. To score a higher percentage than you did for the check-in exercises, try using the chunking method and Number-Association System when suggested. Are you ready to chunk and use your number-images?

14: Airport pick-up

You are a chauffeur working for an international company. You are asked to pick up 4 clients from the airport who are arriving from different cities around the world. Memorize the 4 flight numbers so that you can check the arrivals board at the airport. Try using the Number-Association System. When you are done, cover up the numbers and solve the riddle in the time-lag box. Afterward, try to recall the flight numbers.

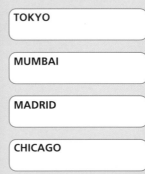

What can bring back the dead, make us cry, make us laugh, make us young? It's born in an instant and lasts a lifetime.

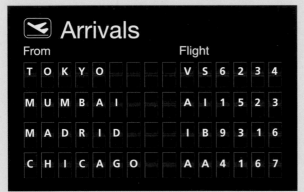

✈ Arrivals

From	Flight
T O K Y O	V S 6 2 3 4
M U M B A I	A I 1 5 2 3
M A D R I D	I B 9 3 1 6
C H I C A G O	A A 4 1 6 7

TOKYO

MUMBAI

MADRID

CHICAGO

Your score: ____
2 points for each flight number recalled

15: Speed demons

The speed of light and the speed of sound are two terms that have become part of our daily parlance, but do you know what the actual speeds are? Well, now is your chance to memorize these numbers. You may want to chunk the numbers. Once you're done, cover up the numbers and take a 5-minute break. Afterward, return to the exercise and try to recall the speeds.

Speed of light =
186,282 mi/sec

Speed of sound =
1,126 ft/sec

Sound

Light

Your score: ____
1 speed: 2 points
2 speeds: 4 points

16: Banking details

A part of your job involves communicating with banks abroad. To do so, you need to memorize the codes that identify these banks. Let's say that the two banks you communicate with the most are identified by the codes written below. Memorize these using the chunking method. When you are done, cover up the codes and find your way through the maze. Afterward, recall the codes.

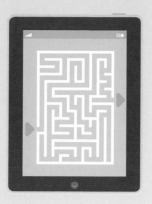

▶ **A:**

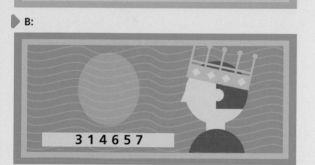

2 0 6 9 8 7

A:

▶ **B:**

3 1 4 6 5 7

B:

Your score: ____
1 code: 2 points
2 codes: 4 points

Solutions on p.185

17: Friendly neighbors

You are having a friendly chat with a couple of ladies at the local café, and during the conversation you discover that they live in a street close to yours. Use the Number-Association System to memorize their house numbers. When you are done, cover up the numbers and, on a separate sheet of paper, list as many different types of cakes as you can think of in 2 minutes. Afterward, try to recall the house numbers.

▶ **A:**   ▶ **B:**

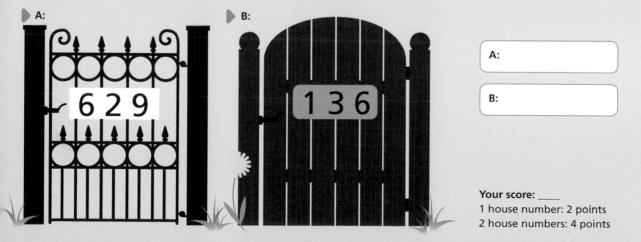

6 2 9   1 3 6

A:

B:

Your score: ____
1 house number: 2 points
2 house numbers: 4 points

18: Online library

Here is your new library access number. Instead of having to refer to your library card every time you request a book online, how about using the chunking method to memorize the number? When you are done, cover it up and try to answer the question in the time-lag box. You have 1 minute. Afterward, try to recall the number.

839208490

Can you name an English word that has three consecutive double letters?

_____

Your score: _____
3+ errors: 2 points
1–2 errors: 4 points
no errors: 5 points

19: Eventful years

Below is a list of years in which a significant event occurred. Try using the Number-Association System to memorize each year and event. When you are done, cover up the dates and, on a separate sheet of paper, take 2 minutes to recall a significant event in your life. Afterward, write down the year next to the picture relating to the event.

1886: The prototype recipe of Coca-Cola is created.

1940: John Lennon, founding member of The Beatles, is born.

1964: The Rolling Stones arrive in New York to begin their first tour in the US.

1969: Neil Armstrong becomes the first man to set foot on the Moon.

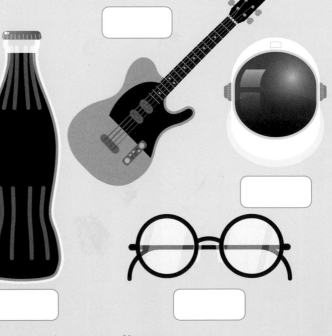

Your score: _____
2 points for each year recalled correctly

20: Sophie's new number

Your granddaughter calls to give you her new phone number. Will you be able to memorize it? See if chunking helps. When you are done, cover up the phone number and, on a separate sheet of paper, list as many childhood friends as you can remember in 2 minutes. Afterward, try to recall the number.

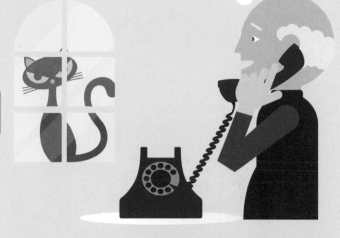

6 1 7 7 4 5 4 9 7 7

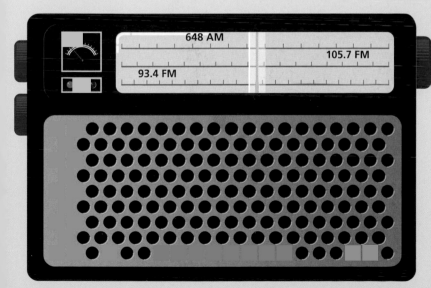

Your score: _____
3+ errors: 2 points
1–2 errors: 4 points
no errors: 5 points

21: Tuning in

Do you sometimes find it difficult to remember the frequency of radio stations? The Number-Association System may be useful here: try it with these 3 radio stations. When you are done, cover up the frequencies and solve the analogies in the time-lag box. Afterward, try to recall the numbers of each frequency.

A: Wolf is to pack as tree is to _____
B: Cat is to kitten as plant is to _____
C: Spin is to dizzy as fire is to _____

648 AM

105.7 FM

93.4 FM

Your score: _____
1 frequency: 2 points
2 frequencies: 4 points
3 frequencies: 6 points

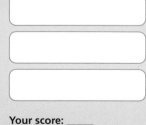

Solutions on p.185

22: Uncle Fred's area code

Uncle Fred has moved to California. Can you memorize his new ZIP code? Use the chunking method to give the number more meaning. When you are done, cover up the number and solve the riddle in the time-lag box. Afterward, recall the ZIP code.

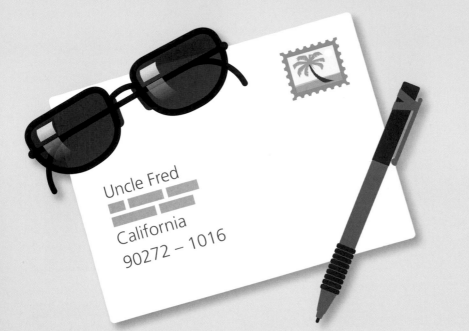

Uncle Fred

California
90272 – 1016

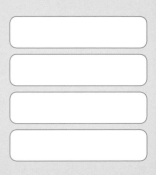

What always runs but never walks, often murmurs, never talks, has a bed but never sleeps, has a mouth but never eats? _____

Your score: _____
3+ errors: 2 points
1–2 errors: 4 points
no errors: 5 points

23: Card verification

During regular online security checks on credit cards, the system often asks for the last 4 digits of the card number instead of the whole series. So it's wise to memorize these digits. Let's practice with the 4-digit numbers below. You may want to use the Number-Association System to boost your memory of them. When you are ready, cover up the numbers and take a 5-minute break. Afterward, try to recall the 4 numbers.

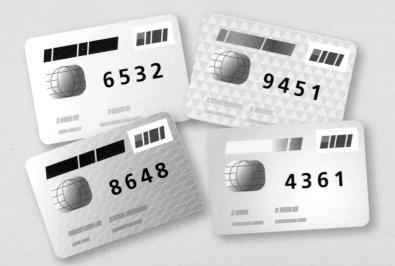

6532

9451

8648

4361

Your score: _____
1–2 card numbers: 2 points
3 card numbers: 4 points
4 card numbers: 6 points

24: Utility bill

Below is your account number for paying the water bill. Can you try to memorize it? See if the chunking method helps. When you are done, cover it up and figure out in the time-lag box what the 5 objects overlapping each other are. Afterward, try to recall the number.

25: Eating cake

Try to memorize the number of calories in each cake pictured below using the Number-Association System. Then cover up the information and take a 2-minute break. Afterward, fill in the calorie figure for each cake.

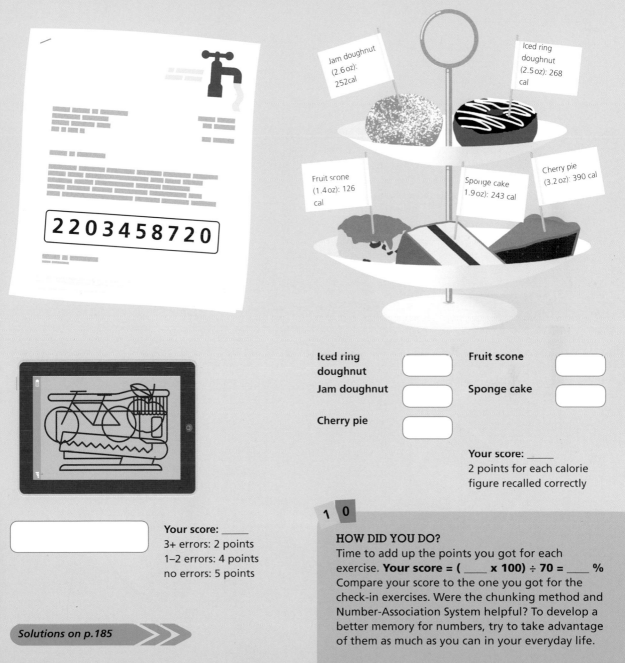

2203458720

Jam doughnut (2.6 oz): 252 cal

Iced ring doughnut (2.5 oz): 268 cal

Fruit scone (1.4 oz): 126 cal

Sponge cake 1.9 oz): 243 cal

Cherry pie (3.2 oz): 390 cal

Iced ring doughnut		**Fruit scone**	
Jam doughnut		**Sponge cake**	
Cherry pie			

Your score: _____
2 points for each calorie figure recalled correctly

1 0

Your score: _____
3+ errors: 2 points
1–2 errors: 4 points
no errors: 5 points

HOW DID YOU DO?
Time to add up the points you got for each exercise. **Your score = (_____ x 100) ÷ 70 = _____ %** Compare your score to the one you got for the check-in exercises. Were the chunking method and Number-Association System helpful? To develop a better memory for numbers, try to take advantage of them as much as you can in your everyday life.

Solutions on p.185

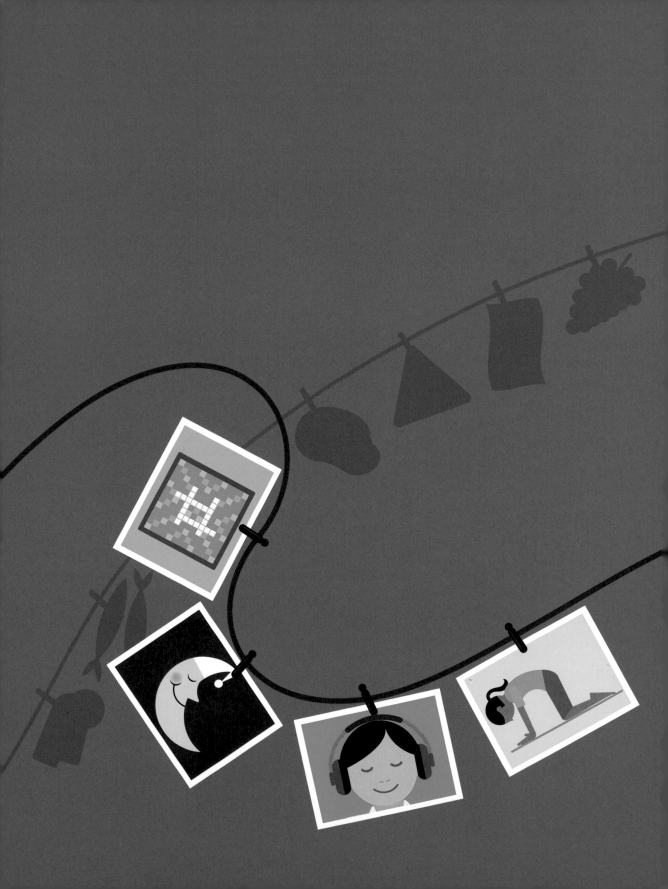

CHAPTER 8
OPTIMIZING YOUR BODY AND MIND (HEALTH AND MEMORY)

It's not what it once was! Does age affect memory?

It's true that some brain functions, such as the working memory, slow down with age. We become more prone to distractions, too, which makes it harder to focus and register information in our long-term memory. Although still sound, our processing power might lose some of its zip. However, by taking more time and minimizing distractions, we can perform to the same level as we used to.

The aging brain

Is it possible to tell which brain is younger by comparing scans of a teenager's brain and the brain of an elderly person? Probably, yes. The older brain is likely to show the general wear and tear that comes from a lifetime of living. In particular, it may be smaller due to some atrophy. Closer observation may also show that the production of neurotransmitters (the chemicals transmitting information between nerve cells) has decreased. Having said that, some people's brains do not show such signs. In fact, individual differences can be quite extreme when it comes to how the brain deals with aging.

Lifestyle choices

Our lifestyle impacts greatly on how our brains and memories age. This is because of "neuroplasticity" (see pp.22–23). Some things are good for brain health while other things are bad, and the extent to which your brain function remains sound throughout life depends partly on your lifestyle choices. The major things you can do to maintain a good memory is eat a balanced diet, manage stress, and exercise both mind and body on a regular basis.

1: It's on the tip of my tongue

Does the correct word sometimes elude you during a conversation? This phenomenon tends to become more frequent as we age. There is nothing pathological about it: in fact, relaxing and ignoring the issue is usually enough to bring the correct word back to mind only moments later. For now, let's assess how easily words come to you (also called your verbal fluency). Write down as many words as possible that may fall under each heading below. You have 1 minute for each. Use a separate sheet of paper if you need more space.

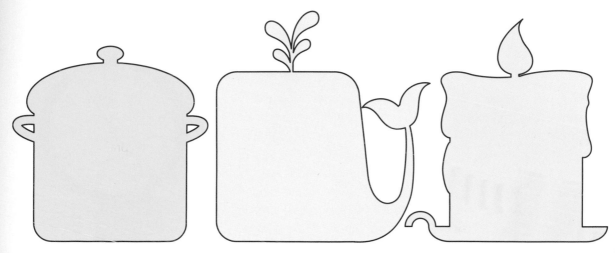

Kitchen equipment   **Sea creatures**   **Fairy tales**

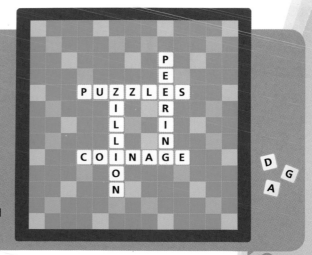

DID YOU KNOW: A LIFESTYLE TO REMEMBER
Do you enjoy playing board games, card games, and crossword puzzles? Do you read newspapers, magazines, or books on a regular basis? Do you like listening to the radio, visiting museums, participating in discussions? Are you educated to a high level? Did you or do you have an intellectually demanding job? Answering yes to any of these questions means that you have a greater chance of maintaining your memory functions and having a resilient brain as you age. Indeed, it seems that the more people participate in activities that engage and stimulate their brain, the better their brain ages.

I'm losing my mind! How to manage stress

Sometimes you just have too much to do and not enough time. On top of that, you seem to be losing your mind: you become overwhelmed, frustrated, and begin forgetting things. Your memory is like a sieve! Does this sound familiar?

The importance of stress

Regardless of whether it is caused by tight deadlines, work overload, or an anxiety to succeed, pressure induces stress. Too much stress is likely to cause memory lapses, irrespective of age. An increase in stress is the body's way of reacting when it senses danger, be it physical or psychological. Stress helps us take flight when we feel a physical threat, or keeps us on our toes when we engage in a high-pressure task, such as giving a presentation to a large audience. Stress triggers the release of stress hormones in the blood: epinephrine and cortisol. These hormones prepare the body for action as the heart starts pumping faster and the muscles tighten up.

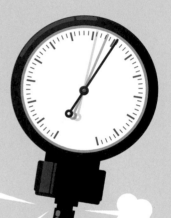

Too much stress!

We've mentioned the positive effects of stress, when stress is occasional. However, chronic stress has negative effects on both your body and mind. It results in lowered immunity response and higher blood pressure. At the level of the brain, it can kill brain cells in regions supporting learning and memory, such as the hippocampus (see pp.14–15). Stress management should therefore be part of any good brain and memory maintenance and enhancement program. Relaxation (through meditation or yoga), physical exercise, and socializing with friends are ways to lower stress. Complete the exercise on the next page to become familiar with meditation techniques.

2: Meditate for your brain health

Most meditation techniques fall into 3 major categories. One is the "open monitoring meditation," which is a type of practice in which you actively pay attention to what is happening inside you, but without reacting or judging. Another is "self-transcending meditation," in which you try to go beyond your own mental activity to reach a restful but alert state of consciousness. Finally, there is "controlled focus meditation" in which you focus attention on your breath, an idea, an image, or emotion. Are you ready to give meditation a try?

Let's start by rating your current stress level:
For each of the body parts depicted on the right, rate how relaxed it is on a scale of 1 to 4 under the "before" heading. (1 = very relaxed, 2 = quite relaxed, 3 = quite tense, and 4 = very tense)

Now follow these steps to enter a relaxed meditative state:
• Find a quiet spot where you can sit or lie down. Close your eyes.
• Take slow, deep breaths. Think about the rhythm of your breathing.
• Relax your body. Focus on each part of your body (start at the feet and work upward) and relax each muscle until it feels heavy.
• Empty your mind. If negative thoughts or distractions come up, ignore them.
• After approximately 15 minutes, allow thoughts to return, but keep your eyes closed.
• Finally, open your eyes and stay seated for a few more minutes before getting up.
• Now rate your stress level again under the "after" heading.

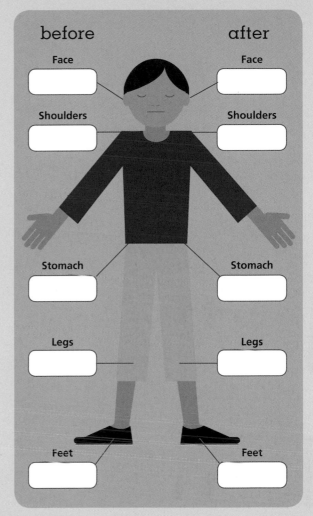

before   after

Face   Face

Shoulders   Shoulders

Stomach   Stomach

Legs   Legs

Feet   Feet

Did it work? Is your overall score lower now? As you probably noticed, it is not always easy to empty your mind. To counter this, you may want to choose a sound ("om"), a word, or a phrase that means something important to you, which you can repeat quietly to yourself during the exercise.

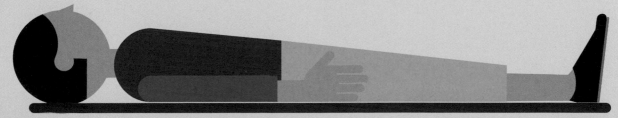

De-stress with yoga

Yoga is a physical, mental, and spiritual discipline that is more than 5,000 years old. The word *yoga* means "to join or yoke together," and the practice is all about finding harmony between the body, mind, and spirit. Yoga involves movement, breathing, and meditation. Its goal is to improve both physical and mental health. There are many different types of yoga. The most commonly practiced is known as *Hatha* Yoga, which includes physical postures and movements as well as breathing techniques.

Yoga poses

Below are three poses to help you relax. Yoga is suitable for most adults of any age, but is not recommended for pregnant women. If you have not exercised in a while, it's advisable to go slowly. If you are not sure, you may want to check with your doctor first, especially if you suffer from back pain or a chronic injury to the wrists or knees.

3: Accomplished pose

This is a very popular seated position for meditation, which is easier than the famous Lotus pose. It opens the hips and lengthens the spine.

• Sit down on the floor with your legs extended. (It will probably be more comfortable if you use a yoga mat.)
• Bend the right knee and tuck the leg underneath you so that the heel presses against your bottom. Keep the knee on the floor.
• Bend the left knee and rest the outside of the left foot behind the right knee so that the left ankle is over the right ankle. The heel of the left foot should line up approximately with the navel.
• Rest your hands on your knees with the palms facing up and the index finger and thumb of each hand touching one another.
• Keep your spine straight and your head up, roll your shoulders back, and push your chest out.
• Relax your face and belly, and breathe. Hold the pose for as long as you feel comfortable.

4: Table pose

This pose is a starting point for other poses, such as the
Cat Tilt pose (see below). It helps stretch and realign the
spine.
• Start on all fours with your knees hip-width apart and
your toes pointing behind you.
• Your hands are directly under your shoulders with your
fingers spread wide.
• Keep your neck long and aligned with your spine and
look several inches in front of you.
• Do not arch or round your back.
• Hold the pose for 5 to 10 breaths.

5: Cat Tilt pose

This pose stretches the shoulders and the middle to
upper back.
• From the Table pose, exhale and tuck your tailbone
under while rounding your spine.
• Let your head drop down.
• Press your palms on the ground to move your
shoulders away from your ears.
• Raise your middle and upper back up toward
the ceiling.
• Hold for 5 to 10 breaths.
• To release, inhale and relax back into the Table pose.

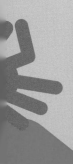

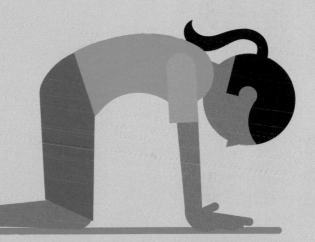

HOW IT WORKS: HOW DOES YOGA HELP RELIEVE STRESS? Research
shows that yoga increases the level of gamma-aminobutyric acid (GABA),
a chemical in the brain that regulates the activity of neurons. Depression
and anxiety are typically associated with low GABA levels, while increased
levels are associated with improved mood and decreased anxiety. A study
showed that practicing yoga for one hour three times a week for 12
weeks improved mood and decreased anxiety more than a comparable
amount of walking. Another study showed that in experienced yoga
practitioners, GABA levels increased by 27 percent after a one-hour yoga
session. In contrast, such an increase was not recorded after an hour of reading.

The importance of sleep

It's a simple matter of fact that sleep deprivation impairs memory and judgment. In contrast, a good night's sleep can improve your memory for what you learned yesterday, what you have to do today, and how to do things (procedural memory, see pp.60–61). This then begs the question as to what goes on inside your brain while you are sleeping?

The different stages of sleep

During a typical night, you go through four to six cycles of sleep. Each cycle is made up of four non-REM sleep stages followed by one REM sleep stage. Here is what a typical cycle looks like:

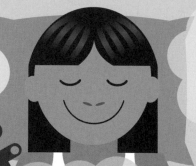

Stage 1 You are falling asleep. It is a light form of sleep from which you can be easily woken. Your brain begins producing theta waves (sleep waves), which are much slower than beta and alpha waves (waves while you are awake).

Stage 3 You are in deep sleep. Your breathing and heart rate are slow and regular. Your brain now also produces low-frequency delta waves. These are often referred to as slow sleep waves.

REM Stage You are still sleeping but your body temperature, and heart and breathing rates, increase. Your eyes move under closed lids and your limbs are temporarily paralyzed. Alpha and beta waves are present in addition to theta waves. You are likely to be dreaming (although you can also dream during non-REM stages).

Stage 2 You are now asleep, but can still be easily woken. Your eyes stop moving. Your body temperature, your heart rate, and your blood pressure drop. Theta waves are still present.

Stage 4 You are now in a state of very deep sleep. It is difficult to wake you up. Delta waves are present.

Brain maintenance during sleep

Although research is ongoing as to how sleep affects memory, what we do know is that during sleep the brain seems to be refueling, organizing information, and discarding what it regards as being irrelevant. Some connections between neurons (see pp.14–15) are eliminated while others are strengthened. Indeed, the processes by which memories become stable may be occurring while we sleep, culminating in the consolidation of memory.

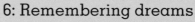

Interestingly, different types of memory may be consolidated during different stages of sleep. For instance, REM sleep may play a role in consolidating "how-to" memories (how to play the violin, for example). In contrast, non-REM sleep stage 3 has been linked to the consolidation of spatial memories. Non-REM sleep stage 4 may play a role in enhancing verbal memories.

How do we know this? Well, boosting the slow sleep waves during non-REM stages (by passing a weak current via electrodes through the scalp) increases the recall of words learned before falling asleep. Also, brain scans of subjects have revealed the same pattern of brain activity occurring during REM sleep as during the learning of a motor task the day before.

6: Remembering dreams

So far, there is no definitive answer as to why we dream. Nevertheless, dreams are usually fun to talk about (as long as you can remember what you dream about). A good way of remembering dreams is to keep a dream diary. Leave the diary close to your bed so that you can write down what you remember as soon as you wake up. See whether what happens to you, or what you experience during that week, has any bearing on the things you dream about.

TOP TIP: A GOOD NIGHT'S SLEEP Here are a few pointers to help you fall asleep and sleep soundly through the night:
• Avoid any caffeine, alcohol, or nicotine before bedtime.
• Do not eat a heavy meal before bedtime.
• Avoid strenuous physical activity (other than sex) within three hours of bedtime.
• Do not stay in bed for too long if you cannot fall asleep. Get up, do something relaxing, such as read a book (not a textbook), meditate, or listen to soothing music, and then try again when you start to feel a little drowsy.

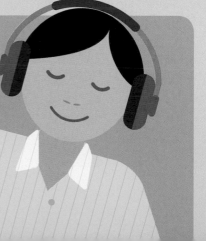

Foods to sharpen your thinking

While it's necessary to feed our brain specific nutrients so that it functions to its highest potential, it's important to choose the right foods so that we absorb a good balance of nutrients. Let's see what's good for the brain and what's bad.

The GOOD

Omega-3 and omega-6

The membranes of brain cells as well as the protective substance that covers them are composed of polyunsaturated fatty acid molecules, such as omega-3 and -6. This explains why you probably have heard these names being associated with brain health and development. Our body doesn't manufacture omega-3 and -6, so we need to get them from our diet. A healthy diet contains a balance of the two fatty acids. Unfortunately, most North Americans and Europeans now get far too much of the omega-6s and not enough of the omega-3s.

• Omega-3 fatty acids are found in cold-water fish (salmon, sardines, mackerel, tuna, and trout) and in some seeds and nuts (flax seeds, chia seeds, and walnuts).
• Omega-6 fatty acids are found in seeds and nuts and the oils extracted from them (sunflower, corn, soy, and sesame oils).

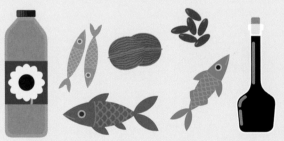

Antioxidants

Antioxidants are molecules that prevent free radicals from damaging cells in our bodies, and this includes brain cells. Free radicals can be formed during oxidation, which is when oxygen interacts with other molecules inside the body. Free radicals can also enter the body via other sources, such as cigarette smoke, pollution, and pesticides. They trigger destructive chain reactions that antioxidants can stop. Fortunately, antioxidants (such as vitamins C and E and many other substances) can be found in a variety of foods, which include:

• Vegetables: spinach, artichoke, avocado, beans
• Dark-skinned fruits and berries: grapes, raisins, blueberries, blackberries, strawberries, raspberries, plums, acai berries, red grapes, cherries
• Nuts: almonds, pecans, walnuts
• Red wine, green tea, fruit juices
• Dark chocolate.

The BAD

Trans and saturated fats

These are not essential to our diet. In fact, consuming too much can increase the risk of cardiovascular disease (and thus Alzheimer's disease) by raising levels of "bad" LDL cholesterol and lowering levels of "good" HDL cholesterol. Trans fats are found in dairy products, meat, butter, and spreads. They are generally used in fast food, snacks, fried food, and baked products as well as many packaged foods. Anything fried has trans fats. Products containing saturated fats include dairy products, meat, eggs, chocolate, and nuts as well as some oils (coconut oil, palm oil, and palm kernel oil).

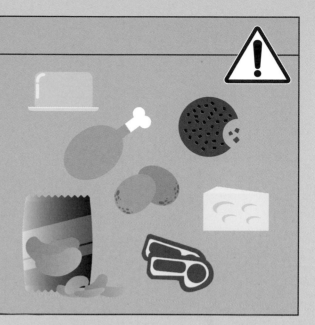

7: The best diet?

There is a diet that offers a healthy balance between omega-3 and omega-6 fatty acids. Studies have shown that people who follow this diet are less likely to develop heart disease and are at lower risk of cognitive decline. What is this diet? The clue's in the picture.

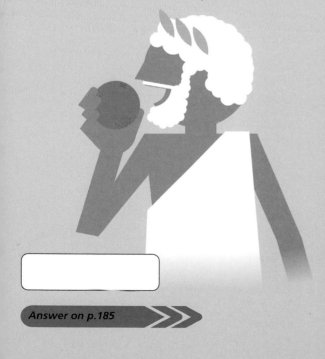

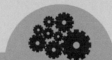

Answer on p.185 >>>

HOW IT WORKS: THE CAFFEINE HIT! Caffeine is a stimulant; it belongs to a chemical group called xanthine. When you drink coffee, your body falsely recognizes caffeine as adenosine, which is a naturally occurring xanthine in the brain that slows down the activity of brain cells (neurons). The caffeine is used by some neurons in place of adenosine. The result is that these neurons speed up instead of slowing down. This increased neuronal activity triggers the release of the epinephrine hormone, which affects your body in several ways: your heartbeat increases, your blood pressure rises, your breathing tubes open up, and sugar is released into the bloodstream for extra energy. Whether this results in increased brain performance is unclear. Studies show contradictory results. Scientists are equally uncertain as to whether caffeine offers any protective effect against age-related cognitive decline.

Exercise to jog the memory

It's no secret that physical exercise keeps the body healthy. But did you know that it also boosts your brain functions? Increasing evidence shows that exercise enhances the brain's performance and protects it from disease and natural decline.

How does it work?

Exercise triggers neuroplastic changes in the brain. Indeed, the volume of some brain regions, specifically regions associated with memory and learning (such as the hippocampus and the frontal lobes), can increase after a period of regular exercise. Studies on animals give us clues as to how exercise may cause this increase in volume. Exercise seems to enhance the production of growth hormones such as BDNF (brain-derived neurotrophic factor). This triggers both neurogenesis (the production of new brain cells) and angiogenesis (the development of new blood vessels). BDNF also helps neurons survive and plays a role in the biological processes associated with the consolidation of memory. In addition, exercise increases the levels of some neurotransmitters such as serotonin (see pp.14–15), thereby helping the transmission of information between neurons.

The best exercise

Aerobic exercise has been repeatedly shown to influence the brain's performance. Aerobic exercise is the kind of exercise that increases your heart rate over a sustained period of time, such as walking, jogging, swimming, bicycling, or dancing.

Of course, you have to exercise regularly to reap the benefits. Guidelines recommend moderate exercise for 30 minutes, three times a week at least. Note that more intense exercise for shorter periods of time, or less strenuous exercise for longer periods of time, work just as well. Usually, you can experience positive and long-lasting effects on the brain about six months into the training. New evidence suggests that resistance and strength physical training (such as using free weights and exercise machines at the gym) for 60 minutes a week can also improve brain function.

The good news is that it is never too late to start exercising and benefiting from it. Age should not be a concern and neither should you worry if you've never exercised before. You just need to find the type of exercise that suits you and begin at an intensity that you find comfortable.

8: Exercise outside the gym

It is not always easy to find the time to go to the gym. Can you list at least 6 ways you can exercise physically during your day at home, at work, or your place of study?

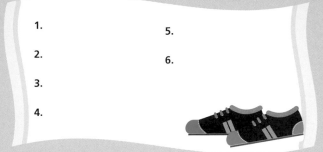

1.
2.
3.
4.
5.
6.

Answers on p.185 ⟫

9: Your aerobic routine

Here is a 10–minute (1 minute per move) aerobic routine to de-stress! You can do it anywhere. Increasing the duration and pace of the movement and adding arm movements will increase the intensity of the exercise. If you have not exercised in a while or if you are unsure, check with your doctor before doing this routine.

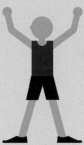
Warm up first: stretch arms and legs then march on the spot

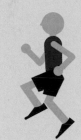
Start jogging on the spot

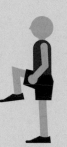
Lift one knee, then the other, and repeat

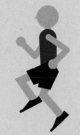
Return to jogging on the spot

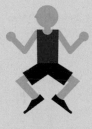
Jump up and down

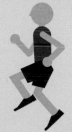
Jog on the spot again

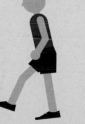
Step forward with your right leg, bring your foot back next to your left foot. Repeat with the left leg. Increase the pace

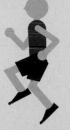
Return to jogging on the spot, gradually slowing down

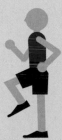
March in place until your heart rate slows down

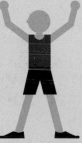
Stretch arms and legs

DID YOU KNOW: EXERCISE DEVELOPS BRAIN AGILITY In a study, 7- to 11-year-old overweight children who enrolled on a 14-week exercise program showed improved brain functions and better performance in mathematical tasks after completing the program. The exercise program resulted in increased activity in the frontal regions of their brains. This study goes some way toward proving that children who play sports at school, take part in other "active" extracurricular activities, or merely enjoy a game of catch after school, appear to reap greater neurological benefit than previously thought.

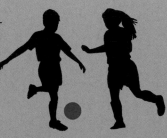

The final word

So now you know some of the most effective ways to improve your memory and keep it in good shape throughout your life. You are also armed with the knowledge to optimize your brain health. If you continue to practice what you have learned in this book, you are definitely on the road to success.

Key things to remember

• Take advantage of your brain plasticity by using your memory on a daily basis. This will ensure that the brain areas supporting memory remain stimulated and potentially improve over time.

• When you are trying to memorize or learn anything, remember that attention, curiosity, and motivation are the natural triggers that can boost your ability to register the material.

• Memory-enhancing techniques have proven their efficacy on many occasions. As you've learned, the majority of these techniques ask you to order information and translate it into memorable images.

• To keep your brain and memory in good shape, it's important to pay attention to your general physical health: clean up your diet, do physical exercise regularly, get adequate amounts of sleep, and try to manage your level of stress.

Summary chart

Use the chart opposite to select the technique(s) that best fits the material you are trying to memorize. Practice using these on a regular basis and soon you will marvel at your growing memory power!

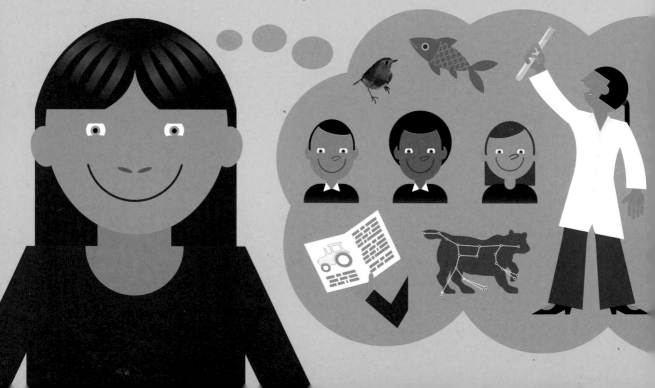

✔ Material to learn/remember	✔ Technique/strategy to use
Names and faces	*The 3-Step Memory Booster (pp.136–137)*
Numbers (phone number, PINs, dates, and so on)	*The chunking method (pp.152–153)* *The Number-Association System (pp.154–155)* *The song method (pp.86–87)* *The major system (p.155)*
Any short list of items (1–5 items on a shopping or to-do list, simple recipe, and so on) **Random pieces of information** (historical events, names of clouds, birds' names, and so on)	*The Link System (pp.88–89)* *The song method (pp.86–87)* *The ordering method (pp.110–111 and pp.112–113)*
Any long list of items (5+ items on a shopping or to-do list, names of constellations, elements of Periodic table, an itinerary of activities, and so on)	*The Journey Method (pp.92–93)* *The Peg System (pp.114–115)*
Extensive amounts of information (a speech, material for a test, instructions to operate a complex machine, a long recipe, details of a project, and so on)	*Mind Webs (pp.118–119)* *The ordering method (pp.110–111 and pp.112–113)*

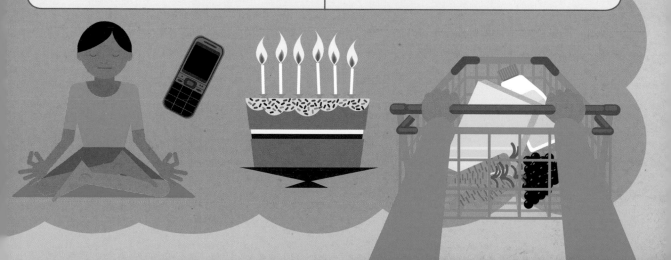

Solutions

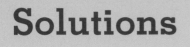 **Chapter 1**

3: It's a matter of size

A: No (Trumpet)
B: Yes (Mobile phone)
C: Yes (Automatic digital camera)
D: No (Handsaw)
E: No (Violin)
F: Yes (Teacup)
G: Yes (Paint brush)
H: No (Drum)
I: No (Saxophone)

4: Label the brain

A: Parietal lobe
B: Occipital lobe
C: Temporal lobe
D: Frontal lobe
E: Hippocampus
F: Limbic system

12: Final destination

B: Meadow Close

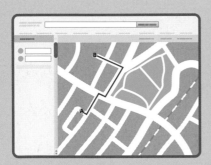

13: The memory quiz

1: B	**6:** A	**11:** B
2: A	**7:** B	**12:** C
3: A	**8:** B	**13:** A
4: C	**9:** A	**14:** A
5: C	**10:** B	

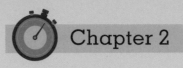 **Chapter 2**

4: Cat invasion!

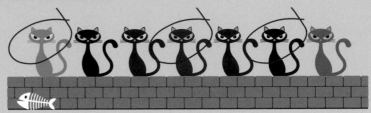

5: Write on your mental screen

Divide 120 by 3 = 40
Divide 125 by 5 = 25
Divide 46 by 2 = 23
Divide 96 by 6 = 16
Divide 300 by 12 = 25
Divide 140 by 4 = 35

12: Mental rotation

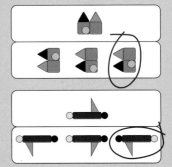

14: Find the odd one out

A:

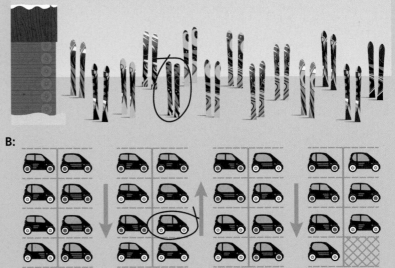

B:

15: Spot the difference

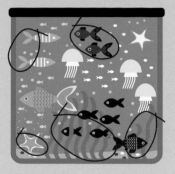

22: Mental drawing

A:

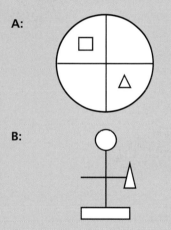

B:

23. Alien visit

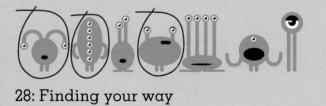

28: Finding your way

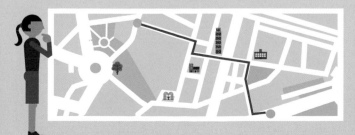

Chapter 3

2: Dining with the famous

Greta Garbo—Hollywood actress
Muhammad Ali—Heavyweight boxing champion
Marie Curie—Physicist & Chemist (Nobel prize winner)
Cleopatra—Ruler of Ancient Egypt
Oprah Winfrey—US chat show host and actress
Mahatma Gandhi—Political and spiritual leader of India
JK Rowling—Author of the Harry Potter books
Isaac Newton—Physicist

3: Visual memories

A: 4 wings
B: Yes. It's approximately 3¼ in
C: 3 arrowheads
D: Left hand
E: 12 inches
F: Red, white, and blue
G: Approximately 1 in

13: It's mine!

Time-lag task:
$(44 + 9) - (23 + 6) = 24$
$(20 \times 3) - (36 - 9) = 33$
$(5 \times 8) - (35 \div 7) = 35$

17: Panic at the toy store!

Time-lag task:
$46 - 14 = 32$
$10 - (4 \times 2) = 2$
$23 + 3 - 9 = 17$
$(5 \times 8) - (5 \times 4) = 20$

18: Martian invasion

Latest headline: a large Martian **sighting** is confirmed. The first spacecrafts were **spotted** this **morning** over Spain and France. Further reports indicate that the fleet is heading toward Great **Britain**. In London, the streets are filling up with **worried** citizens gazing at the sky. **Supermarkets** are full as people are trying to buy anything they can before the invasion. Cars and **buses** are lining up on the main **roads**. Traveling may become **difficult** in a few hours.

20: Facing the enemies

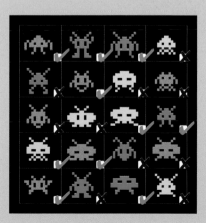

Time-lag task:
BATTLE
ENVELOPE
CHICKEN
COMPUTER

21: Eyewitness
A: Guitar
B: Stroller
C: No
D: 10 lamps
E: Leaning against a lamppost
F: No
G: Cane
H: 10 people

Time-lag task:
$(10 \times 7) - 45 = 25$
$(6 \times 10) + (9 + 9) = 78$
$(7 \times 4) - (15 \times 0) = 28$
$(86 - 74) + (9 \times 3) = 39$

22: Reading a map

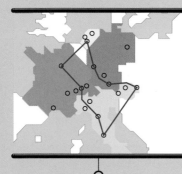

26: Birthday wish
Time-lag task:

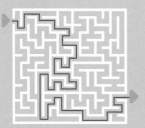

27: Follow the recipe

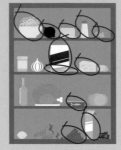

Time-lag task:
424.4° Fahrenheit

28: Geography lesson

River	Ocean
Mississippi	Gulf of Mexico
Jordan	Dead Sea
Seine	English Channel
Ganges	Indian Ocean
Danube	Black Sea
Euphrates	Persian Gulf
Amazon	Atlantic Ocean
Mekong	South China Sea

Chapter 4

4: Mental scale
A: DVD case: Smaller
B: Mobile phone: Larger
C: Checkbook: Larger
D: Ballpoint pen: Larger
E: Wine bottle: Smaller
F: Cotton swab: Larger
G: Fork: Smaller
H: Coffee mug: Smaller
I: Business card: Larger

6: Imaginary turns
A: Identical
B: Mirrored
C: Identical
D: Mirrored
E: Identical
F: Mirrored

7: It's all in the detail
A: Short tails
B: Yellow/orange
C: No, the tip of the beak and parts of the outer wing are black.
D: White/gray
E: Large ears
F: A boot

10: Funny images
Objects: lion, cage, ostrich, toothbrush, towel, bench, man, book, tree, frog, horse, green fence, scissors, hand, pink cat, cookies, glass of milk, red and white straw, plate.
Time-lag task:
$(60 \times 3) + (90 - 30) = 240$
$(30 \times 4) - (36 - 10) = 94$
$(24 + 9) + (8 \times 2) = 49$

23: Memorize to music
Time-lag task:
The nail in a horseshoe
Footsteps

25: The wedding speech
Time-lag task
$(120 \times 3) - (25 \times 2) + 54 = 364$
$(80 + 26) + (23 \times 3) - 45 = 130$

26: Does it fit in a shoebox?
Coat hanger: No
Colander: No
Hair dryer: Yes
Cereal box: No
Tambourine: No
Child's doll: Yes
Table tennis paddle: Yes
Bicycle pump: Yes
Laptop: No
Ice skates: No

30: Cube folding
Answer: C

Chapter 5

1: Accessories

For women: lipstick, perfume, purse
For men: dumbbell, top hat, wallet
For children: ball, slingshot, teddy bear

2: Ranking game

By size (small to large): diamond ring, calculator, telephone, vase, umbrella, laptop computer, car
By value: umbrella, vase, calculator, telephone, laptop computer, car, diamond ring

3: What's on my kitchen table?

Table A
1. 6 dairy products: cheese, milk, yogurt, ice cream, butter, cream
2. 6 meats: sausage, steak, chicken, pork, turkey, lamb
3. 6 vegetables: corn, potato, bean, carrot, broccoli, leek

Table B
1. 5 orange-colored fruit/ vegetable: apricot, pumpkin, orange, tangerine, carrot
2. 5 red-colored fruit/vegetable: strawberry, cherry, tomato, radish, raspberry
3. 5 green-colored fruit/ vegetable: zucchini, spinach, peas, lettuce, artichoke

4: Going fishing

There are 4 species:
1. Tail type 1
2. Tail type 2
3. Blunt fins
4. Pronounced gills

5: Who are they?

Soccer player: soccer ball, soccer ball boots, pair of shorts
Artist: coloring pencils, sheet of paper, easel, paint set, ruler
Scientist: test tube, protective goggles, latex gloves, microscope

6: Slide puzzle

The picture depicts the first moon landing in 1969.

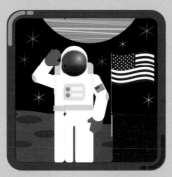

7: Up for grabs

1: Objects that make a sound when they're used: telephone, violin, baby's rattle, radio, bell, trumpet
2: Objects that do not make a sound when they're used: scissors, cup, pencil, book, sunglasses, bottle

8: Sorting shapes

First ordering system: colors of the rainbow
Second ordering system: number of sides in ascending order
Third ordering system: number of dots in ascending order

9: What belongs where?

The 4 categories are:
Vehicles (private modes of transportation); Vehicles (public modes of transportation); Facial features; Other body parts

12: Weekend shopping

Hardware store: paint brush, masking tape, light switch
Chemist: cough drops, cotton balls, nail polish, bandages, vitamin pills
Garden center: potting soil, flower seeds, rake, watering can

14: Let's go shopping

Time-lag task:
$(125 + 41) - (8 \times 2) = 150$
$(12 \times 6) + (71 + 28) = 171$
$(23 + 26) + (15 \times 4) = 109$
$(52 + 20) - (9 \times 8) = 0$

19: A trove of toys

Meaningful categories:
Sports equipment: soccer ball, badminton racket, cricket bat, shuttlecock
Toy vehicles: coach, train, jeep, tractor
Cuddly animal toys: teddy bear, panda, penguin, lion

20: The coldest places on Earth

Time-lag task:
$(12 \times 6) - (4 + 12) = 56$
$(5 \times 8) + (7 - 5) = 42$
$(60 \div 4) + (26 - 12) = 29$

21: Ring fingers

The rings can be grouped by the shape of their stone (circular, square, rectangular), or by color (red: ruby, green: emerald, and blue: sapphire).

Time-lag task:
Answer: False

25: Cloud gazer

Organization principle: cloud levels
Low clouds: stratus, nimbostratus, cumulus,
Middle clouds: altostratus, stratocumulus, altocumulus
High clouds: cirrostratus, cirrus, cirrus-cumulus
Exception: Cumulonimbus

Time-lag task:
12 + 15 + 6 + 9 + 11 − 30 + 8 = 31
6 − 3 + 8 + 17 − 9 + 22 + 5 = 46

28: Decathlon
Time-lag task:
(230 − 90) + (15 x 4) = 200
(124 − 12) + (8 x 6) − (45 + 9) = 106

29: Fixing the house

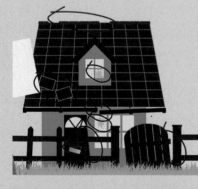

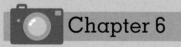

Chapter 6

2: New bank workers

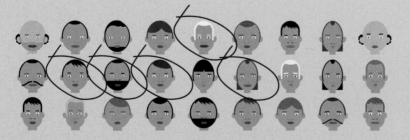

4: Observing faces

A: Light brown
B: Yes
C: No
D: No
E: Yes
F: A flat nose

5: Back to the bank

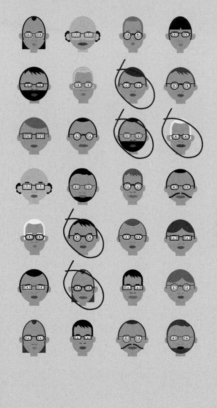

8: On a day trip

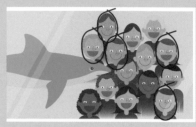

Time-lag task:
26 + 51 + 32 + 64 = 173
43 + 31 + 36 − 20 = 90
34 + 45 + 7 − 21 = 65
32 + 12 − 30 + 11 = 25

11: The new batch

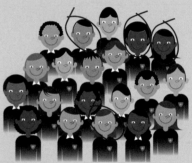

14: Meet the teachers

A: Yes
B: Biology
C: Mrs. Reed
D: No
E: No
F: Ms. Crawford

15: Friends of a friend
Time-lag task:
Answer: C elastic

17: Business relations
Time-lag task:
(45 x 3) + (32 + 56) = 223
(35 ÷ 7) x (42 − 6) = 180
(21 − 6) + (7 x 8) = 71
(6 x 12) − (23 − 7) = 56

18: Too many docs!

Time-lag task:

1: Be attentive to boost memory (pp.40–41)
2: Basic principles to improve memory for the past (pp.62–63)
3: The Link System (pp.88–89)
4: The Journey Method (pp.92–93)
5: The Peg System (pp.114–115)
6: Mental Maps (pp.118–119)
7: The 3-step memory booster (pp.136–137)

19: On first-name terms

Time-lag task:

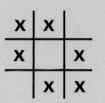

20: Party time!

Time-lag task:
67 + 45 − 6 = 106
34 + 4 − 8 = 30
23 − 7 + 26 = 42
424 − 234 = 190

Chapter 7

4: Important phone number

Time-lag task:
Answer: Your name

5: Code to enter the site

Time-lag task:

Answer: Give the 4 children an apple each and then give the last child the basket with the apple in it.

6: Age is just a number

Time-lag task:

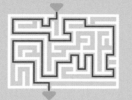

7: Knitwear for Christmas

Time-lag task:
3 x left turns
3 x right turns

10: A slice of pi

Time-lag task:
Answer: Charcoal

12: Birth years

Time-lag task:
Carrot
Strawberry
Cantaloupe

13: Safe delivery

Time-lag task
Answer: Stars

14: Airport pick up

Time-lag task
Answer: A memory

16: Banking details

Time-lag task:

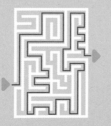

18: Online library

Time-lag task:
Answer: Bookkeeper

21: Tuning in

Time-lag task:
A: Forest
B: Sapling
C: Hot

22: Uncle Fred's area code

Time-lag task:
Answer: A river

24: Utility bill

Time-lag task:

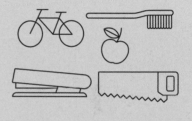

Chapter 8

7: The best diet

The Mediterranean diet. This diet does not include much meat. The emphasis is on whole grains, fresh fruits and vegetables, fish, olive oil, garlic, as well as a moderate amount of wine.

8: Exercise outside the gym

1: Always take the stairs instead of elevators
2: Park you car farther than you normally would from your destination
3: Take a walk outside during your lunch break
4: Put on some music in the house and dance to it
5: Do some gardening
6: Housework (vacuuming the house offers a good physical workout)

Useful websites

GENERAL INFORMATION ON MEMORY

www.sharpbrains.com

www.dana.org

www.pbs.org/wnet/brain/

www.youramazingbrain.org/yourmemory/

www.improvememory.org

www.waystoimprovememory.com

www.memorise.org

www.memory-loss.org

www.gloo.com.au

MORE PUZZLES AND FURTHER INFORMATION

Short-term memory

www.fupa.com/play/Puzzles-free-games/short-term-memory

www.free-sudoku-puzzles.com/games/memory-game/short-term-memory-game.php

www.onlinegamescastle.com/game/short-term-memory

www.everydayhealth.com/longevity/mental-fitness/brain-exercises-for-memory.aspx

Long-term memory

www.lumosity.com

www.toimprovememory.com/longtermmemoryactivities.php

www.memoryjoggingpuzzles.com

Memory and imagination

www.enchantedmind.com/html/science/creative_memory.html

www.cul.co.uk/creative/puzzles.htm

www.supplementsformemorytips.com/Improve-Memory-When-You-Improve-Creativity.html

Memory and organization

www.web-us.com/memory/improving_memory.htm

www.npmanagement.org/Article_List/Articles/Organizational_Memory.htm

Remembering names and faces

www.memory-key.com/improving/strategies/everyday/remembering-names-faces

www.howtoimprovememory.org/names-faces/

www.mymemoryfix.com/remember_faces.html

Remembering numbers

www.braingle.com/mind/test_numbers.php

www.improvememory.org/how-to-improve-memory/memorization-techniques-remember-numbers

www.memorise.org/lesson3.htm
(For further information about the Major System)

Your body and mind

www.learningmeditation.com
(For more information on meditation)

National Institutes of Health
http://health.nih.gov
(Advice on symptoms of stress, treatment, and prevention)

The World Health Organization
www.who.int/occupational_health/topics/stressatwp/en/
www.cdc.gov/niosh/topics/stress
(Advice on stress at the workplace)

The British Wheel of Yoga
www.bwy.org.uk
(Find a certified yoga teacher anywhere in the world)

Further reading

Introduction to the brain
Searching for memory: The Brain, the Mind, and the Past by Daniel L. Schacter (Basic books), 1997

Learning and Memory: The Brain in Action by Marilee B. Sprenger (ASCD), 2003

The Rough Guide to the Brain by Barry Gibb (Rough Guides), 2007

The Human Brain: A Guided Tour by Susan Greenfield (Phoenix), 2001

Memory improving techniques and exercises
Don't Forget: Easy Exercises for a Better Memory by Danielle C. Lapp (DeCapo Press), 1995

Intelligent Memory: Exercise Your Mind and Make Yourself Smarter by Barry Gordon and Lisa Berger (Vermilion,) 2003

How to Develop a Brilliant Memory Week by Week: 52 Proven Ways to Enhance Your Memory Skills by Dominic O'Brien (Duncan Baird Publishers), 2005

Intelligent Memory by Barry Gordon and Lisa Berger (Vermilion), 2003

Exercises in Memory by Frank Channing Haddock (Kessinger Publishing), 2010

Maximize Your Memory: Techniques and Exercises for Remembering Just about Anything by Jonathan Hancock (Reader's Digest Association), 2000

Memory and creativity
Cognition: From Memory to Creativity by Robert W. Weisberg and Lauretta M. Reeves (John Wiley & Sons), 2012

The Mind Map Book: Unlock Your Creativity, Boost Your Memory, Change Your Life by Tony Buzan (BBC Active), 2009

Brainpower: Practical Ways to Boost Your Memory, Creativity and Thinking Capacity by Laureli Blyth (Barnes & Noble Books), 2002

Memory and health
Saving Your Brain: The Revolutionary Plan to Boost Brain Power, Improve Memory and Protect Yourself Against Aging and Alzheimer's by Jeffrey Ivan Victoroff (Bantum Doubleday Dell), 2004

How to Improve Memory and Brain Function as we Age by Parris Kidd (Keats Pub Inc.),1997

Yoga Mind, Body and Spirit: A Return to Wholeness by Donna Farhi (Newleaf), 2001

How to Activate Your Brain: A Practical Guide Book by Valentin Bragin M.D Ph.D (AuthorHouse), 2007

Super Body, Super Brain: The Workout That Does it All by Michael Gonzalez-Wallace (HarperOne), 2011

General
The Sharp Brains Guide to Brain Fitness: 18 Interviews with Scientists, Practical Advice, and Product Reviews, to Keep Your Brain Sharp by Alvaro Fernandez & Dr. Elkhonon Goldberg (Sharpbrains, Incorporated), 2009

My Stroke of Insight: A Brain Scientist's Personal Journey by Jill Bolte Taylor (Hodder), 2009

The Brain That Changes Itself: Stories of Personal Triumph from the Frontiers of Brain by Norman Doidge Science (Penguin), 2007

Spark: The Revolutionary New Science of Exercise and the Brain by John J. Ratey and Eric Hagerman (Quercus Publishing), 2008

The Memory Book: The Classic Guide to Improving Your Memory at Work, at School, and at Play by Harry Lorayne and Jerry Lucas (Ballantine Books), 1986

Index

About the Author

Dr. Pascale Michelon

Pascale Michelon is a research scientist at Washington University in the Pycology department. Dr. Michelon's passion for applying and sharing scientific knowledge led her into the field of brain fitness and memory improvement. She has worked with both young and older adults to understand how the brain processes information and memorizes facts. In 2006, she founded The Memory Practice to provide adults with challenging cognitive exercises to keep their brain fit. Dr. Michelon has received several academic fellowships and awards. From 2004 to 2006, she received the Washington University Center for Aging award for her research into the effects of aging on spatial reasoning. Dr. Michelon is also an Expert Contributor for the website SharpBrains.com, where individuals, companies, and institutions are provided with the best science-based information and guidance on brain health and fitness.

Acknowledgments

Author's acknowledgments

I would like to start by thanking my editor Suhel Ahmed for his thoughtful support, his rapid and enlightening feedback, and his enthusiasm for the project from start to finish. I would like to thank Keith Hagan for his fresh, colorful, and striking illustration, without which this book would clearly not be the same. Many thanks to Charlotte Seymour for overseeing every aspect of the book's design, and my gratitude also goes to Nicola Erdpresser who did a fantastic job of marrying the text and illustrations: it was always a pleasure to see the proofs during the book's production. Thanks also to Angela Baynham for her solid editorial work.

Finally, I would like to thank my family and particularly Pascal, for his continued support and his complete trust in my projects and dreams.

Publisher's acknowledgments

DK Publishing would like to thank Hillary Bird for supplying the index and Alyson Silverwood for proofreading the book in such a short amount of time. Also, many thanks to them and their families for checking the puzzles and exercises.

We would like to extend our thanks to Giles Smith, the marketing manager at **www.travelindependent.info**, for providing us access to their online entry for South America on pp.120–121

Picture Credits

The publisher would like to thank the following for their kind permission to reproduce their photographs: (Key: a-above; b-below/bottom; c-centre; f-far; l-left; r-right; t-top)

16 John Foxx: (cr). **Getty Images:** Digital Vision (cra); Stockbyte (ca). **59 Getty Images:** McDaniel Woolf (ftr). **133 Getty Images:** Monica Lau (ca). **Imagestate:** (c, fcr, cl). **138 John Foxx:** (crb). **Imagestate:** (cr, cra, br). **141 John Foxx:** (bc, fbl, bl). **Getty Images:** C. Borland / PhotoLink (cb); Monica Lau (clb). **Inmagine:** (cl). **142 Imagestate:** (cl). **145 Getty Images:** Don Tremain (c). **150 Imagestate:** (br)

All other images © Dorling Kindersley
For further information see: www.dkimages.com